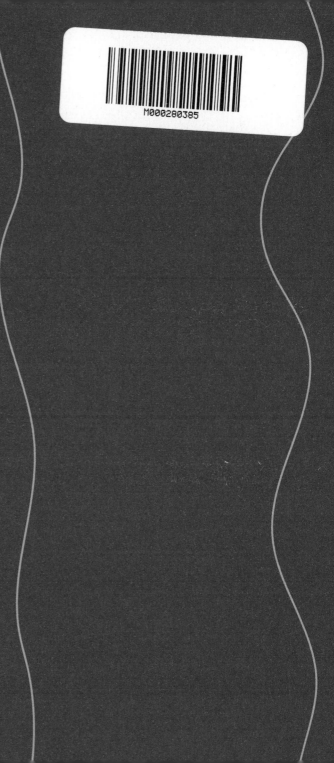

Rest Easy

Rest Easy

DISCOVER CALM and ABUNDANCE through the RADICAL POWER of REST

XIMENA VENGOECHEA

Foreword by Alexandra Elle

CHRONICLE BOOKS

SAN FRANCISCO

Library of Congress Cataloging-in-Publication Data available.

ISBN 978-1-7972-1947-9

Manufactured in China.

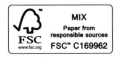

Design by Wynne Au-Yeung.
Typeset in Albra, Baskerville, and TT Norms.

Some names and identifying details have been changed
to protect the privacy of individuals.

10 9 8 7 6 5 4 3 2 1

Chronicle books and gifts are available at special quantity
discounts to corporations, professional associations, literacy
programs, and other organizations. For details and discount
information, please contact our premiums department at
corporatesales@chroniclebooks.com or at 1-800-759-0190.

Chronicle Books LLC
680 Second Street
San Francisco, California 94107
www.chroniclebooks.com

FOR ISAAC

Contents

Foreword

As someone who works in the healing space, I've come to see that rest and healing are intertwined. They need each other. When we need to heal anything, be it a physical ailment, like a broken bone, or an emotional ailment, like a broken heart, we need to rest. We need to take a moment, to press pause, to put our feet up, to commit to our restoration.

Unfortunately, we don't live in a world that encourages us to rest, which is why it's so important to have tools like *Rest Easy* that help us create ease in our lives. As you'll see in these pages, there are so many ways to rest our minds, our bodies, and our spirits. Rest is personal; we each have to find what works best for us, to keep us filled up and energized. I've come to understand that emotional rest really fuels me. When I give myself a chance to rest emotionally and when I take a step back to connect with my true feelings and set healthy boundaries, I am reminded that I don't have to solve everything today.

When we rest, we have the power to shift generational cycles of exhaustion. I've seen the people in my lineage—especially the women— do things on very little rest, and it's not sustainable. By resting, I am breaking cycles. By resting, I am setting aside intentional space for slowing down. By resting, I am making space for joy, for presence, and for doing absolutely nothing.

The more people talk about resting and being present and doing nothing, the more we start to dismantle the systems that keep us from resting and the more we start to normalize taking things slow and giving ourselves space to get clear on things without rushing. The more we rest, the more we disprove the idea that we have to always be doing something. The more we rest, the more we get to know ourselves.

Imagine how remarkable and how magnificent it would be if more of us were rested. To do that, we need to discover how to rest in ways that make us feel safe and supported. *Rest Easy* invites you to look at your life and to look at where you're resting, where you're not, and where you need to create the space to care for yourself. It reminds us to slow down, to be present, and to stop always doing. It invites you to take intentional pauses to get still, get clear, and be open to what's in front of you so that you can enjoy a nourished, abundant life.

—ALEXANDRA ELLE, *New York Times*
bestselling author of *How We Heal*

The Power of Rest

My mother says I came out of the womb with a notebook under my arm. I was a perpetually organized child, self-disciplined and focused—the kind of kid who, according to family lore, planned her own birthday party at age five because otherwise it wouldn't get done.

To be laser focused on getting things done is both a blessing and a curse—it has made me a highly productive, and therefore valued, member of our capitalist society. But it has also left me exhausted. If I can't relax until I get through my responsibilities, well, I'll never get to relax at all. And I'm not alone.

While researching and writing this book, I heard from hundreds of people experiencing a chronic rest deficit. I heard stories from Elena, a young nurse who lived by the motto "Work hard, play hard," but knew her lifestyle had become unsustainable when she started napping in her office closet. And Daniela, a sales consultant who worked long hours and was often on the road for work. "I'll sleep when I'm dead," she boasted to friends. Until one day when she nearly fell asleep behind the wheel. She knew then that something had to change.

Some people see the signs early on that a break is needed. They are tired, so they sleep instead of caffeinating. They are disagreeable, so they journal to understand their emotions instead of remaining angry at the world. They notice when their energy flags, their mood changes, and their motivation wanes and listlessness sets in. They listen. They accept. They rest.

But some of us don't. Like Elena and Daniela, some of us learned a long time ago to ignore the signs that it's time to slow down. We keep going because we believe ourselves unstoppable, or because life's responsibilities—work, rent, or kids—make it impossible to stop. Sometimes we press on because deep down we actually enjoy being busy—we feel the pride and exhilaration of living intensely, the seductive and powerful pull of checking things off our to-do lists.

A World Craving Rest

Today, many of us struggle to get the rest we need. My generation, millennials, are particularly susceptible to the overwhelm. We entered the job market in the wake of a crumbling economy. Many of us are plagued with memories of the Great Recession, when being a hard worker wasn't enough to secure a job (much less keep one). Some of us used this time to hide out in graduate school, often taking on loans that still haunt us today. Others sought out more entrepreneurial ventures—as gig workers, start-uppers, side-project hustlers, and members of the creator economy. Wherever we landed, we worked our tails off. When the specter of job loss hangs over you, doing anything less than 110 percent can feel dangerous. It's no wonder that, in recent years, we have embraced movements like quiet quitting—treating your job like a job, not a vocation—as we get deeper into adulthood.

Of course, this isn't just a millennial problem, or an American problem either—although it is in peak form in the United States, as evidenced in movements such as FIRE (Financial Independence, Retire Early), #vanlife, and the Great Resignation. In Hong Kong, you can pay to take a "sleeping bus tour," which offers a five-hour, 47-mile (76-kilometer) route so exhausted residents can get some shut-eye. (Tickets include an eye mask and earplugs.) In China, the tang ping, or "lying flat," movement has taken hold among young workers, who are quitting their jobs in record numbers in order to "lie down" and rest. Theirs is a quiet protest of a work culture that frequently expects employees to work twelve-hour days, six days a week. Other Chinese workers partake in an activity that has resonated worldwide, "revenge bedtime procrastination"—putting off sleep at the end of a long day in order to get leisure time in, which unfortunately makes us more tired than before. In Japan, death by overwork, or karoshi, is a known problem. Research from the World Health Organization shows that death by overwork has spread beyond Japan's borders, and it suggests that anyone working long hours (more than fifty-five a week) is at increased risk of heart disease and stroke. Across cultures, we see a desperate need for more rest and relaxation.

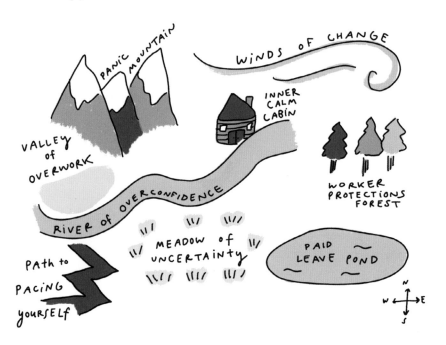

MAPPING OUR Emotional LANDSCAPE

Whether it's work, parenting, pet care, marriage maintenance, elder care, erranding, or bill paying, the list of responsibilities on our plates is daunting. Add to the mix a twisted backdrop of job insecurity, climate disaster, political unrest, social and racial injustice, and pandemic anxiety, and it's no wonder so many of us are overwhelmed. As we will learn, our cultural values, religious beliefs, economic circumstances, national histories, and personalities all play a role in how seriously we take the problem of rest.

Breakpoint

While researching this book, I came across many stories of accomplished individuals who crashed and burned in spectacular fashion. Academic and activist Dr. Devon Price suffered from anemia and heart complications from overexertion. Yoga teacher Octavia Raheem was hospitalized with rhabdomyolysis after overworking her body. Dr. Elizabeth Stanley, now an army veteran and professor at Georgetown, found herself vomiting on her computer after clocking sixteen-hour days while working on her PhD.

My come-to-Jesus moment was far less dramatic. I never wound up in the ER or a doctor's office (although my therapist certainly heard a lot from me those days). Mine was a slow burn—insidious and perhaps even a bit dull—but it was life changing. Sometimes it doesn't take a storied catastrophe to turn us around. Sometimes it's death by a thousand paper cuts.

I knew something had to change in the fall of 2020, when I was offered the role of a lifetime. I'd been hanging by a thread while working three jobs: one at a top tech company with a toxic work environment, another as a debut author, and another as a new mother. In between my newborn's cries and naps, I wrote my first book, tried to keep my team happy, and ran employee-resource groups for other women struggling like me. Friends were impressed I could juggle so much, but in truth, I was like a duck swimming around in circles—graceful on the surface, but paddling furiously beneath the water, and on the verge of drowning.

When the pandemic hit, my strategy of simply putting one foot in front of the other began to crumble. I remember discussing with my therapist whether I could hold on just a little bit longer to see the new role through. I was exhausted, but surely, I thought, I could do it.

Two weeks into my new role, I found myself unexcited, unmotivated, and even more tired than before. I knew I should feel grateful—the role had been tailor-made for me—but all I felt was dread. I dragged my feet on making plans and setting goals. I mustered fake enthusiasm for a job I realized I no longer cared for. What was the point? I felt apathetic about what happened next; I simply didn't have the energy for it.

Finally, I did what I should have done years before: I quit my tech job. Thanks to my partner's stable job and the savings I'd built since my first job as a teen reporter, I could afford to leave my nine-to-five. I'd be back on the job market in no time, I told myself. I would take a month off, six weeks at most. Surely, I'd feel like myself by then.

Quitting was my first rest experiment—a personal experiment and a means to regaining my energy. But it didn't take long for me to realize the disconnect between my vision and my reality. In quitting, I did not unearth a magic source of energy waiting to be tapped. I was still the same tired me, only now without a job. (Yikes.) Though I was glad to have a break from the office politics and aggressive deadlines, and I eventually started to feel a *little* less overwhelmed, it was no silver bullet.

Reclaiming Realistic Rest

Most people cannot afford the luxury of voluntarily removing themselves from the workforce and taking an unfunded sabbatical. And as my experience showed, even the lucky few among us who can do this still struggle to recover from feeling depleted. As the days ticked by, I realized that I didn't know *how* to bounce back from my exhaustion. I had no idea what concrete steps to take to feel rested. All I knew, it seemed, was how to work.

I was familiar with the mainstream advice for how to encourage rest (exercise, get eight hours of sleep a night, take naps, set devices aside before going to bed, meditate, and so on). Some of that advice felt completely out of reach, especially as the mother of a toddler not yet in daycare. (Naps? For me? Hilarious.) Others I stubbornly resisted (I have a hate-hate relationship with exercise, so anything more strenuous than a brisk walk or scenic hike was hardly appealing). Conventional wisdom is often broad and easy to follow in theory, but hardly motivating.

People told me to "slow down," "take it easy," "relax," and "stress less"—but no one could tell me what that looked like. The assumption, it seemed, was that resting meant not working (maybe even not moving), but given my experience on "sabbatical," that didn't seem right. Everyone I knew could tell me what a good work ethic looked like, but hardly anyone could advise me on cultivating a good rest ethic. People said structural change was needed (agreed!)—but it also seemed unlikely to change during my lifetime. How was I to manage in the meantime?

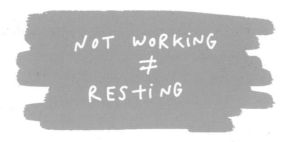

I wanted to know: Which activities are *actually* restorative, and which are overhyped? Why do we sometimes self-sabotage our efforts to rest? Is it really possible to slow down without feeling guilty? What can we ask of others—our families, employers, and governments—to make our quest for rest more within reach? When I couldn't find the answers on Google or Amazon (kidding, kind of), I decided to take matters into my own hands.

This is the story of how I learned to rest. Or, rather, the story of how I, in my very type-A way, systematically uncovered the key ingredients for getting high-quality rest. In order to uncover the secret to good rest, I've talked to experts, read a ton, crowdsourced insights from everyday aspiring resters like me and you, and conducted a series of personal experiments to uncover the best resting tactics to incorporate into your world. The stories, insights, and rest practices you read about in this book are a distillation of this work. I'm your human guinea pig, your guide, and your supporter as you work to get the rest you deserve.

WhAt WE thiNK of AS RESt

ANotheR NigHt of MiNDLESS StREAMiNg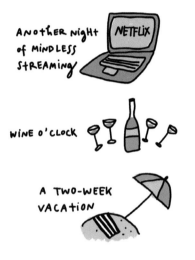

WiNE O'CLOCK

A TWO-WEEK VACAtiON

WhAt RESt ActuALLy iS

PuzzLES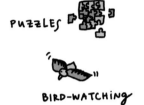

BIRD-WATCHiNg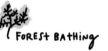

FoRESt BAthiNg   WHitE NOiSE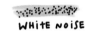

A TWO-MiNutE MEDiTATiON

PLAy

In chapter 1, we'll look at the science and psychology behind why rest is so important—for our mind, body, and spirit. In chapter 2, we'll explore common cultural, systemic, and societal blockers we may face in our quest for rest, and in chapter 3, we'll look at the ways we may hold *ourselves* back from rest. Later, in chapter 4, we'll learn real, actionable techniques for resting, and in chapter 5, we'll learn how to design our own personal rest routine. By the end of the book, you will have the right tools to get the rest you need, along with some final encouragement and advice to get started.

Throughout the book you'll also find a series of sidebars designed to help you deepen your rest practice. These include

> **Self-reflect:** Questions to help you build awareness of your unique circumstances, preferences, and obstacles so that you can thoughtfully design a rest practice that works for you.

> **Take a Micro-Moment of Rest:** Short sidebars that feature brief exercises to help you get the rest you need now, in five minutes or less.

> **Deepen Your Rest Practice:** Exercises to help you further strengthen your rest practice when you have time to spare. I've tested each one of these myself, so you can trust I've picked only the best for you.

> **Take Note:** Quick facts and illuminating insights from my rest research to inspire you on your rest journey.

The practices I've shared throughout the book are based on the following criteria:

o **Easy.** We are all busy. Personally, the more difficult a technique is, the more likely I am to ignore, resist, and ultimately reject it—and you may be the same. I designed this book with people like us in mind. If a technique was too complicated, it didn't make the cut.

o **Affordable (mostly free).** Cost can be a barrier to getting rest, so I wrote this book with budget-friendly options in mind. You won't get stuck buying scented candles, incense kits, weighted blankets, and other "stuff" you might not need.

- ○ **Enjoyable.** Rest should be pleasant, not a chore. As we'll learn later in the book, when it comes to building new habits, it helps to enjoy yourself.

- ○ **Proven.** It would be easy to get lost in the latest wellness trends without a guidepost or two, so I made sure there were no bold claims without backup here. Rest techniques I included needed to be proven, meaning scientifically backed, evidence-based, or grounded through science, sociology, history, religion, cultural anthropology, psychology, or other fields. This could include clinical trials, but also valuable techniques from alternative medicine where the science hasn't yet caught up (for example, practices such as meditation and breathwork have been widely revered, practiced, and understood in many parts of the world for centuries, yet they have only relatively recently been studied in Western lab settings).

As we'll see, reclaiming rest is an issue of both personal and societal responsibility. Later, I share policy changes that can help us lead more rested lives. But such changes take time. For that reason, I spend the bulk of my time on how you can get through your day-to-day life *today*.

You can read this book cover to cover, or you can hop around as you please. Although I've tried to keep suggestions actionable and accessible, not all advice will be for you. As we'll learn in chapter 2, your individual identity—your race, ethnicity, gender, sexuality, and spirituality, along with whether or not you are a caretaker, among other

Rest Easy

qualities—also affects your ability to rest. Later, we'll see how your unique personality can help or hinder your rest efforts and determine the kind of rest that works best for you. Other circumstances, such as your mental health, will also inform which practices are most useful to you. You know yourself best, so find what works for you and set aside the rest.

As you explore the rest techniques in this book, you might find it helpful to reach out to your doctor, therapist, or others in your support circle if you have questions about which techniques are best suited for you or how to best adapt a technique for your life. Consider this book a starting point for deeper exploration and discussion.

I recommend starting small on implementing new rest practices to help you gain confidence as you find the type of rest that's right for you. Start where there's heat, and if a tactic sounds like a chore, skip it. Once you gain some momentum, you may find you're ready to take on more challenging rest practices from there. Don't feel like you have to take on *all* the advice in this book. If you're like me, that overachieving tendency can be strong. But resting isn't about achievement or competition. Resting well is about going at your own pace and in your own time.

Resting is an essential part of living well: It helps us to be more creative, empathetic, healthy, and, yes, even more productive. Perhaps most importantly, having regular, restorative moments of respite allows us to connect with priorities outside of work, like family, friendship, self, and community. Rest is what enables us to be a person in the world.

You do not need my permission to rest, but I'm going to give it to you anyway. It is normal and healthy to want a break. To want to pause. To want to *be* for a moment, instead of to *do*. That does not make you weak—it makes you human. Rest is not earned or deserved; it is as necessary as food and water. You have permission to sink in slowly and partake.

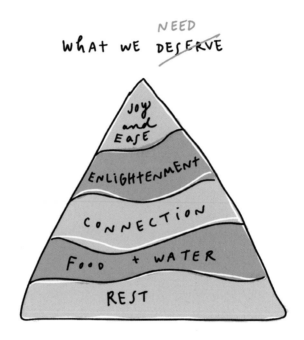

WHAT WE ~~DESERVE~~ NEED

JOY and EASE

ENLIGHTENMENT

CONNECTION

FOOD + WATER

REST

SELF-REFLECT: **What Does Rest Mean to You?**

Take a few minutes to make a list of things that leave you feeling rested and recharged—activities, moments, environments, even people. Aim for five to ten items on your list.

Looking at your list, think about the qualities that make these activities most restful to you. Are they solo activities or done in a group? Who are they with? Are they active or passive? Cerebral or physical? Spiritual or practical? What do you like best about these moments or activities?

Notice any patterns in what you find restful, along with any surprises. For example, perhaps you find that your most restful practices are solo ones, or you are surprised to find that activities that you don't intuitively think of as restful, like running, actually are.

As you explore this book, remember these insights; let them serve as a guide and help you to choose the rest techniques that are right for you.

Chapter 1

The Case

for Rest

WHY REST MATTERS

W e've all pushed ourselves too far at one point or another. Sometimes, circumstances are beyond our control. Prioritizing rest may be too hard, too inconvenient, or too expensive—in time and money. Sometimes it is *ourselves* who get in the way. Unraveling what we've been taught about rest and work takes effort.

Unfortunately, when we fail to get adequate rest, our physical, emotional, and cognitive health and well-being suffer. When fatigue sets in, our patience usually wears thin, and we aren't as kind and compassionate to others as we ought to be. Many of us, when we are burned out and exhausted, become hollow, overworked, overtired shells of people. Everything—including our ability to focus and concentrate, physically recover, and form emotional connections—is at risk when we aren't well rested.

REST BRINGS...	NOT ...
ABUNDANCE	SCARCITY
GENEROSITY	STINGINESS
OPENNESS	CLOSED-MINDEDNESS
GOODWILL	ILL WILL
JOY	SADNESS
LOVE	HATE
EASE	UNEASE
CALM	STRESS
WARMTH	OVERWHELM
LEVITY	DISTANCE

The Magic of Rest

When we are rested, we are able to access a higher version of ourselves. We become more generous partners, kinder colleagues, friendlier neighbors, and better parents and children. We are more patient, empathetic, calm, and joyful. We have goodwill to spare and to spread. We believe others are doing their best, rather than expecting them to disappoint us. We are satisfied by what is possible, rather than frustrated by what is not. We are better equipped to be there for others because we are there for ourselves. We handle life's unexpected ups and downs with grace instead of chaos. We are accepting and loving rather than judging and withholding. We are content with the small moments that make up our days. Rest helps us to reduce stress, but just as crucially, it also helps us to access joy, calm, pleasure, peace, abundance, and connection. Rest is a pathway to feeling like our whole selves.

When we are rested, we tap into self-confidence rather than self-doubt. Energized, inspired, and uplifted, we put our best foot forward and share that self with others. We can be ourselves and accept others as they are too. We are open to learning, to making and admitting mistakes, to being vulnerable. We are present, attentive, openhearted, and creative. When we allow ourselves to *be*, rather than constantly doing or planning, life's little joys and possibilities reveal themselves to us. Our hearts fill and our minds quiet when we nourish ourselves with rest.

In my own life, I know that when I am feeling rested, I can better handle whatever ups and downs come my way, be they toddler tantrums, my Gemini husband's quick mood changes, or a meeting at work that goes awry. I am more flexible and resilient—a better colleague, friend, spouse, daughter, and mother—when I have more gas in the tank.

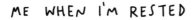

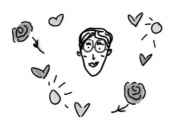 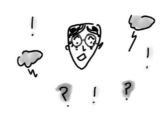

COOL, CALM,   FRANTIC,
COLLECTED,   STRESSED, †
+ LOVING   SHORT - FUSED

What Is Rest?

Despite the benefits, many of us struggle to incorporate rest into our lives. Before we can put rest into practice, we need to understand what it is and how it works.

Rest is a state of being in which nothing is required of us. It is a time where we can just *be*. For some, this will be an active experience— dancing, running, or walking can all be restful, depending on the person. For others, this will primarily be a passive experience, such as reading, sleeping, daydreaming, or drawing. Rest can be mental, physical, or spiritual—or sometimes all three.

Because what's restful for me may not be restful to you, I define rest as any ritual, habit, or activity that makes you feel refreshed, recharged, calm, or at ease. If you are wondering whether an activity is restful, it's probably not. Usually, we know rest when we see or feel it—our bodies relax, our minds quiet, our feelings settle. (Scrolling social media may "look" like rest, but does it leave you energized or at ease?)

THE MANY FLAVORS OF REST

ACTIVE

PASSIVE

SOLO

SOCIAL

CALMING

ENERGIZING

Here are some of the ways people described rest to me. As you read through, think about which sentiments feel truest to you.

PEOPLE DESCRIBE REST AS...

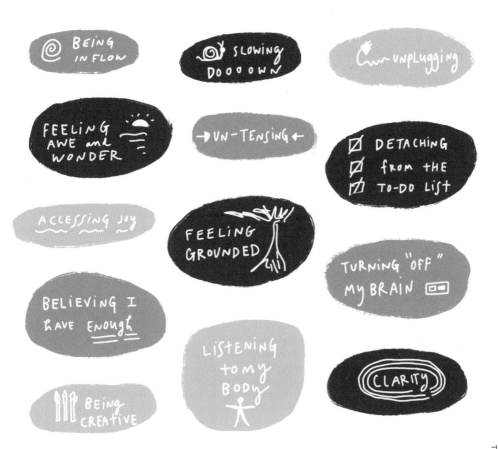

BEING IN FLOW

SLOWING DOOOOWN

UNPLUGGING

FEELING AWE and WONDER

UN-TENSING

☑ DETACHING
☑ from the
☑ TO-DO LiST

ACCESSING JOY

FEELING GROUNDED

TURNING "OFF" MY BRAIN

BELIEVING I HAVE ENOUGH

LISTENING to my BODY

BEING CREATIVE

CLARITY

Three Kinds of Rest

There are three main categories of rest, each of which we'll explore more deeply in chapter 4. Here is a brief overview to get you started.

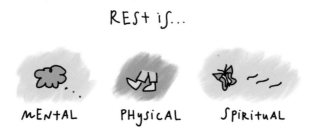

Mental Rest

Why is it that our best ideas come in the shower? It is because our brains are on a break. As often as possible, the brain goes into what is called the default mode—flitting from idea to idea, subconsciously making connections, recalling memories consolidated during sleep, and finding solutions where our own conscious efforts failed. This mode is responsible for gems like self-reflection, introspection, and empathy toward others. The brain excels in this rested state.

Taking breaks allows the mind to do what it does best—wander—and has been shown to make us more creative, healthy, and productive. We can give our brains a boost by spacing out, daydreaming, people watching, and immersing ourselves in art or nature. Mental breaks mean giving the brain a breather from work, social media, and endless to-dos.

When we power through and ignore the need for mental breaks, we don't allow our brains to access this crucial mode. As a result,

Rest Easy

we become prone to decision fatigue, poor decision-making, and decreased performance. It may seem counterintuitive, but resting our attention is an investment in our focus, concentration, problem-solving, and short-term memory.

Physical Rest

Rest is as crucial for the mind as it is for the body. Though we may at times believe, insist, or pretend otherwise, the body requires a pause in order to strengthen and operate maximally. Many elite athletes know that having a "rest day" is crucial for improving one's physical performance, and they honor them religiously.

Restful physical activities like breathing deeply, lying down, or taking a walk in nature have been shown to regulate blood pressure, heart rate, and glucose levels. Sleep—the ultimate pause—is a proven stress reducer and immune-system booster, helping us to repair cells and strengthen neural connections overnight.

Rest is also extremely effective against the wear and tear of chronic stress on the nervous system. When our fight-or-flight system (the sympathetic nervous system) is activated, it needs its opposite, the rest-and-digest system (the parasympathetic nervous system) to help dampen that arousal. "Rest is a huge part of that biological process," says clinical psychologist and stress researcher Dr. Darby Saxbe. "It helps you get back to your set point."

Importantly, how we cope with stress has a big impact on our ability to activate and harness that rest-and-digest mode. "It's not just about having an escape hatch," Saxbe told me in an interview. "It's a mindful or deliberate attempt to recharge and reenter the world, as opposed to pulling away and giving up." How we cope—whether we use *avoidant* coping mechanisms (like turning to substances or screens) or *approaching* coping mechanisms (like problem-solving and seeking social support)— matters. We'll learn more about the best coping mechanisms for managing stress in chapter 4.

Spiritual Rest

It's no surprise that many spiritual experiences—be they grounded in organized religion or experienced in nature—are considered to be restful and restorative. Taking a moment to *be* rather than *do* is at the center of a number of religious traditions—from the Jewish Sabbath and Christianity's Sunday day of rest to the meditative practice of Buddhists. Even those of us who are not religious can connect to a greater wisdom through stillness—by watching the sun set, listening to a breeze ripple through the leaves of a nearby tree, or being in quiet community with others at a coffee shop, concert hall, or other shared space. What is true across these experiences is that it takes a moment—a space, a pause, a quiet, a stillness—to connect with yourself and a greater sense of purpose. We'll explore spiritual and healing practices for rest in more detail in the chapters to come.

What Happens
When We Don't Rest

Here are some common consequences of a lack of rest.

Worker Burnout

According to the World Health Organization, worker burnout results
from unmanaged, chronic workplace stress. Burnout has three parts:
feeling exhausted; feeling distant, cynical, or negative about one's job;
and devaluing and losing confidence in your abilities. In other words,
you're tired, you DGAF, and you're not sure you can do your job well.
To really solve burnout, organizations have to change how they divvy
up work, train workers, and reward workers for their efforts. Ultimately
the organization is what needs fixing, not you. It can be hard to see that
distinction when we're exhausted.

Parental Burnout

According to a 2022 Ohio State University study, 66 percent of working parents are burned out. These parents may feel exhausted, irritable, or emotionally detached from parenting. Many feel overwhelmed and like they have nothing left to give.

Chronic Stress

One of the clearest signs that rest is needed is experiencing chronic stress. When we're chronically stressed, we experience a constant state of fight-or-flight. Our bodies experience this as a lack of safety—we stay vigilant, alert for danger, rather than relaxing. This permanent state of fight-or-flight impairs our memory, distorts our reality (making us more attuned to fear), suppresses our immune function (cue the stress-induced head cold), and even increases our risk for cardiovascular disease.

Activate Your Rest-and-Digest Mode

If you're feeling stressed, try this micro-moment of rest to activate your rest-and-digest mode. According to Dr. Herbert Benson, a pioneer of mind-body medicine and author of *The Relaxation Response*, we can activate our rest-and-digest mode with a few simple steps:

1. Choose a word or phrase you will repeat during this restful practice. For example, you might choose a word like *calm*, *gentle*, *abundance*, or *peace*. This will anchor your practice.

2. Take a seated position, close your eyes, and for two minutes progressively relax your muscles from your toes to your head. On every exhalation, repeat the word or phrase you've chosen. Whenever a thought enters your mind, return to your anchor word.

3. At the end of your session, notice how you feel. Has your heart rate slowed? Do you feel a sense of calm?

If you enjoy this practice, use it to activate your rest mode a few times a day to reduce stress. You might also extend this practice from two minutes to ten and notice how this change impacts your nervous system.

If you find this practice challenging (as I did when I first started), try this bite-size version instead: Simply close your eyes for one minute and listen to the sound of your breath or your surroundings.

Chapter 2

Busyness

Is Bigger than Us

CULTURAL AND SYSTEMIC
BLOCKERS TO REST

As a New Yorker, I am always in a rush. Sure, spending seven years living in Northern California—land of wineries, scenic hikes, and farm-to-table meals—tempered my inner sense of urgency a little bit. But as anyone in my family will tell you, I've always been the impatient type (and I probably always will be).

These days, you don't have to be preternaturally impatient or type A to feel the pressure to move faster. Many of us suffer from hurry sickness. We seem to live in a constant state of fast-forward, propelled by a persistent, overwhelming pressure to do more. We may feel perpetually behind and anxious about all that's left to do. Between often-crushing work expectations and always-on technology that enables us to be reachable even on vacation, it can be hard to slow down and relax. For many of us, being busy feels more like a fact than a choice—an inevitability we must succumb to rather than overcome.

Unfortunately, all of this hurry comes at a cost: We may run ourselves ragged because we consistently fail to prioritize rest. We may lose out on quality time at home because we're too focused on meaningless to-dos, missing the big picture of what's important. With nary a moment to pause, many of us feel disconnected from our loved ones, our purpose, and our communities. "I missed a moment to cuddle with my son today," recalls Nia, a stay-at-home mom and part-time school administrator. "We were at home and he looked so peaceful lounging on the couch. I wanted to lie down with him, but I am just too busy."

Despite the drawbacks of our busyness, many of us find it hard to slow down. In this chapter we'll look at how we got so busy, and the invisible, external forces pushing us to do more and rest less.

FORCES THAT SHAPE OUR
RELATIONSHIP TO REST:

CULTURAL   SYSTEMIC   INDIVIDUAL

We'll look at the cultural and systemic blockers to rest—the stuff that, without us even realizing it, shapes our relationship to work, rest, and play. It's in the food we eat, the air we breathe, the TV we watch, and the magazines we read. It permeates through popular culture and our workplaces, schools, and homes—day by day, drip by drip by drip. Depending on where we live and where we're from, these forces can help or hinder our efforts to rest. (Spoiler alert: It doesn't look good for Americans.)

In the pages to come, we'll dive deep into just what these forces are and how they affect—and sometimes even warp—our relationship with rest. Specifically, we'll look at how cultural views and systemic policies about work, parenting, technology, and identity impact our ability to rest. When we understand what we're up against, we can learn how to manage it and get the rest we need.

TAKE NOTE: **The Busy Badge**

In the nineteenth and early twentieth centuries, leisure time was a highly coveted status symbol. The wealthy used their time to entertain and be entertained—not work themselves to the bone. Leisure was the status symbol, not busyness.

Since then, being busy has become a badge of honor in our society—a way to signal our importance to others—at least for the well-off. But if we dedicate our time to *doing* rather than *being*, we will be hard-pressed to feel relaxed.

Luckily, we are at the beginning of a cultural shift that once more values leisure, rest, and relaxation. Don't miss your chance to be a part of this movement—slow down.

Work

Most of us spend a disproportionate amount of time working and thinking about work. Thanks to inventions and policies old and new, work (and before that, school) is often the activity we spend the largest chunk of our day-to-day time on.

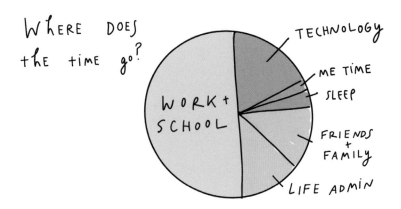

WHERE DOES the time go?

WORK + SCHOOL

TECHNOLOGY

ME TIME

SLEEP

FRIENDS + FAMILY

LIFE ADMIN

Although work and rest are not always diametrically opposed, it frequently feels that way. Because work is tied to our financial security, it can be hard to pull ourselves away from another overtime shift, PowerPoint revision, or email—even when we know it's time to shut down. The shift to remote work has further blurred the lines between work and home; our commutes may be shorter, but our boundaries have become more porous. This is often good for employers' bottom lines, but not always good for the rest of us. Here are some common cultural myths that stop us from resting.

The Virtue of Work

In many societies, and particularly in the United States, work is not just a means to an end (say, a paycheck), but a reflection of our character. Thanks to societal ideologies like the Protestant work ethic, many of us believe that working—and therefore being productive—is a virtue. We respect hard work and dislike (or even fear) idleness and perceived laziness. We may even feel that to work hard is to *be* good—to be worthy of love and all the trappings of a nice life. If we have a good work ethic, we must be deserving. In this view, not working becomes a moral failing, a character defect. Not working means trouble. (As the biblical saying goes, "Idle hands are the devil's workshop.") Not working makes us bad. This explains why so many of us feel guilty, or even ashamed, about not being productive. Unfortunately, viewing leisure as immoral is likely to leave us overworked, overtired, and under-rested. We need to shake this point of view if we are to wholeheartedly reap the benefits of rest.

Hard Work and Hustle

In individualist societies, hard work is not simply a sign of virtue, but a means to greatness. In the United States, for example, the pull-yourself-up-by-your-bootstraps mentality is deeply embedded in the culture and policies. The idea that if you work hard you can make it, no matter who you are or where you come from, reflects an individualistic perspective that you are in control of your own destiny. (This is very different from more communal or collectivist societies, which believe the success of an individual is dependent on the community through shared knowledge, values, and support.)

"My father came to this country in '89 with very little money, so rest was not part of his equation to success," Jenny, a first-generation American and aspiring rester told me. "Growing up, he told me to not rest too much and to not be lazy—hard work does not include lounging around. As Korean immigrants, my dad and mom did not get to rest very often. They always worked hard to provide—to survive, not thrive."

The belief that hard work means that anything is possible is encouraging and is not without its merits. There are many heartwarming stories of people working hard and successfully breaking through class lines to create stable lives for their families.

Yet personalizing success in this way—as the sole result of an individual's efforts—suggests that we *should* be able to do everything on our own. This can lead to a slew of anti-rest behaviors, like not asking for help when we need it or putting our work above taking care of ourselves. The myth that success comes from hard work alone (as opposed to, say, economic, racial, and gender privilege) has led many of us to resent when our minds and bodies tire and demand a break. Because of it, we may have come to mistakenly believe that help, self-care, and rest are the enemies of success, instead of essential ingredients for it.

Love Where You Work

Today, it's not enough to work hard—you have to be passionate about your work too. Cultural (and employer) messages like "love where you work" serve as both advice and command. It's common to be told that we should love our jobs—to be there not just for a paycheck, but for the team (your new "family") and mission. It's expected that if you have a hobby or passion project, you'll monetize it, because who doesn't want to get paid to do what they love?

Unfortunately, loving our jobs inevitably leads us to make certain sacrifices, particularly when it comes to rest. When we love what we do, it is easy to work long hours and think about work even when we are not working—but that doesn't mean we should. Loving our jobs can cause us to lose perspective and get lost in overwork. We can easily forget to stop and play, rest, and explore when we are so single-mindedly focused. We may overlook corporate policies that seem designed with our well-being in mind, but aren't, like the free but frequently late dinners that keep us in the office longer.

When we "do what we love," we often sacrifice our time and money. Creatives like writers and artists are frequently expected to work for little pay (because their work is so meaningful, of course). Teachers and other "mission-driven" workers must also accept a pay cut for their noble work. Many people in these professions end up working multiple jobs to make ends meet, making rest difficult to prioritize. The message that we should love our jobs can make it hard to admit when our jobs don't love us back.

The Pressure to Be Productive

Productivity culture claims that if we can just get our to-do lists and priorities right, we'll finally be able to master our days. Many of us do what we can to check the boxes faster and be more efficient under the assumption that we will get to relax afterward. We can't possibly rest if there's still more to do.

But this is the wrong way to think about it. In fact, becoming more productive usually only makes things worse: The better we get at email, the more emails we get. The faster we complete projects, the more projects we are assigned.

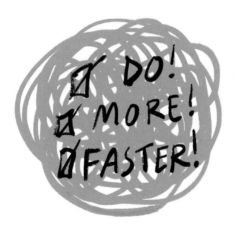

The myth of productivity is that things will eventually get better—that we will reach a promised land where we have accomplished All the Things and are at peace. The reality is that once we are done with one task, another crops up. If we let our urge to be productive take the driver's seat, we'll never get to a rest stop.

TAKE NOTE: **Productivity Dysmorphia**

For some of us, being productive isn't just about trying to check everything off of our list. It's also a way to feel like we are worthy individuals *deserving* of rest and happiness. But tying our self-worth to our output is an unwinnable game. It can get so bad that we no longer recognize our achievements for what they are. Journalist Anna Codrea-Rado coined the term *productivity dysmorphia* to describe the disconnect we sometimes feel between our actual, objective accomplishments and our subjective experience of them. When I published my first book, instead of experiencing it as a major achievement—especially given what I'd sacrificed to write it—I remember immediately thinking, "Done. What's next?" I barely stopped to celebrate and reflect on all the work that went into it.

According to Codrea-Rado, productivity dysmorphia stems from a mix of anxiety, burnout, and imposter syndrome. "How productivity dysmorphia manifests for me is in me feeling that my achievement is not real. But what I'm really saying with that is that this achievement isn't good enough. And that means I am not good enough," she told me. It's particularly common for women and people of color to feel this way, given they are more likely to be undervalued—paid less, promoted less, given less credit for their ideas— within their organizations. It's harder to recognize your efforts when the broader ecosystem doesn't. We'll learn more about how our identity affects our ability to rest later in this chapter.

The Problem of Multitasking

The myth of multitasking is the belief that doing more than one thing at a time is productive—or even possible. The truth is that it is neither of those things. Many of us are expected to juggle multiple tasks at once as part of our workflow, or feel that we must in order to be productive and not fall behind. We may catch up on emails during a meeting, work on a project while listening to a presentation, or respond to a text message during a one-on-one. In these moments, it can feel like we are getting a lot done, but research shows that we're getting less done, and at a lower quality, than we think. Every time we switch between tasks (which is what's *actually* happening when we multitask), we tax the brain, which makes us tired. The more scattered our attention, the more resources the brain needs, and the more fatigued we feel. It's more productive—and restful—to simply focus on one thing at a time.

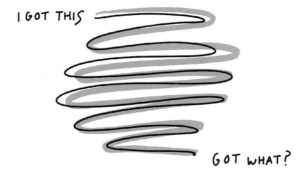

CONTEXT- SWITCHING and the BRAIN

I GOT THIS

GOT WHAT?

TAKE NOTE: **Inspiration from around the World**

Many cultures prioritize leisure and well-being—from France's commitment to lingering over an elaborate meal and Denmark's value of community living to Italy's respect for la dolce vita. These aren't just philosophical mindsets: Many countries have specific policies that make it easier to rest, like limiting the number of hours of work per week (capped at thirty-seven in France) or making it illegal to be contacted by your employer after work hours (as in Portugal).

Below are a few of the ways that countries around the world prioritize their citizens' well-being:

Protected nights and weekends: Several countries, like France, have established "right to disconnect" laws for workers. This gives workers the right to unplug after work hours and during weekends, and forbids employers from expecting work output during those hours. Dreamy!

Required annual time off: France, Spain, Austria, Germany, Canada, and Japan all offer at least twenty days of paid vacation and holidays per year.

Shorter workweeks: Four-day workweek trials have taken place in Spain, Ireland, New Zealand, Scotland, and Iceland. Data from one of the earliest trials, in Iceland, is particularly encouraging—after shortening the workweek from forty hours per week to thirty-five to thirty-six hours per week (with no change in pay), worker well-being increased and productivity improved or stayed the same.

Parenting

Whether you are a full-time, stay-at-home parent or racing to get home from work before bath time every night, parenting is defined by trade-offs. Take care of yourself or take care of your family? Go for the job promotion or lean back and let someone else have a go? Stay late at the office or risk upsetting your boss to get home in time for family dinner? This kind of trade-off thinking is mentally taxing. And rest? Forget about it. It's all hands on deck now.

Becoming a parent is a great privilege, yet it comes at a cost. Many parents throughout the world lack the kind of social support and infra-structure needed to raise their families. American parents, who lack the social support offered in many industrialized countries, like universal childcare, paid family leave, and job protection while on leave—often struggle to balance work and childcare, much less make time for themselves. How can they rest when dinner needs to get on the table, the kids need help with homework, the dog just took a pee on the plants, and the laundry isn't done? This is especially true for families who cannot afford to hire a nanny, chef, or personal assistant (which is most of us).

Adding fuel to the fire are the many cultural pressures that tend to push rest lower on the priority list for parents. From Pinterest-perfect parties to Instagram-ready family portraits, many parents (and especially mothers) are expected to be perfect. Social media tends to edit out the realities of messy rooms and sibling bickering, as well as help from caregivers outside the nuclear family unit. It can be hard not to internalize the cultural messaging that being a good parent means doing everything yourself and holding yourself to unrealistic standards. These attitudes make it more difficult for parents to tend to themselves and rest.

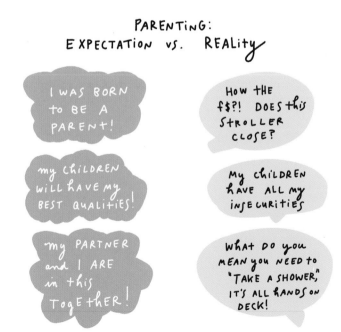

PARENTING:
EXPECTATION vs. REALITY

I WAS BORN to BE A PARENT!

HOW tHE f$?! DOES this StRoLLER cLoSE?

my cHiLDREN wiLL hAVE my BEST QuALitiES!

My cHiLDREN hAVE ALL my inSEcuRitieS

my PARTNER and I ARE in this TogE+hER!

whAt Do you MEAN you NEED to "TAKE A SHOWER," IT'S ALL hANDS oN DECK!

New parents face added stressors. Relationships suffer tremendously during the early years of a child's life—marital satisfaction decreases, while stress levels increase. Statistically speaking, the birth of a first child is even a risk factor for divorce. (For women, divorce can be particularly bleak: They tend to suffer the financial ramifications of divorce the most.) Although many couples believe becoming parents will bring them together, it isn't always (or even often) the case. On top of being anxious about how they will manage their new family responsibilities, they may feel isolated from the support system they need most—their partners. This kind of emotional stress makes recharging all the more essential.

Raising a family can bring many happy memories, but behind every successful science fair, soccer game, playdate, and teachable moment is a tremendous amount of hard work. Yet if we are unable to care for ourselves as we do for our children, we will quickly find ourselves burned out, exhausted, grumpy, and unable to enjoy the company of our children and all the goofy and funny kid things they do. As parents, we need to find ways to lighten our load every day—with help from our communities and institutions—and to embrace the idea that to parent well we need to rest well too.

Technology

There's little to say about technology and its impact on our health, well-being, and ability to rest that hasn't been said already. Research suggests that our smartphones, particularly the social media we view on them, contribute to feelings of loneliness and hinder our sense of community. Merely having a phone visible in a conversation can reduce our empathy toward others as well as our ability to concentrate. Repeated, intermittent screen usage can impair our attention spans, focus, and memory. Time seems to vanish whenever we look at our phones, each (self-)interruption making us feel busier and more behind. Even if you don't know the stats or the science, chances are you feel this in your bones and understand it intuitively.

Despite knowing the downsides, it's very difficult to change our relationship with our devices. As a user researcher at some of the top tech companies in San Francisco, I can confidently say it's not entirely your fault—your attachment to your device is not simply a reflection of your willpower, moral virtues, or discipline. The features we find most addictive on our favorite apps and websites are by design. Notifications give us a little dopamine hit and can offer social validation. News feeds that repopulate in an instant exploit the brain's tendency toward the novel (the novelty effect) and keep us coming back for more, like a slot machine in Vegas. Frictionless, autoplaying videos and reels keep the novelty coming and make it hard to look away. These features capitalize on our desires, cravings, and base impulses. Combined with some very human instincts and needs—to be loved, to be part of a community, to feel like we are in the know, to be validated and affirmed, to be entertained—these features make it hard to step back from our often-toxic relationships with social media, breaking news, and email. Worse, they remove the small, natural pauses in our lives we'd otherwise take to check in on ourselves and others.

I've experimented with many ways to curb my device usage—from turning my phone to gray scale and turning off notifications to "saving" certain apps for web-only usage. I've also scrapped a lot of suggestions that sound great in theory but are difficult to put into practice. Many of those, like reserving a dedicated hour per day for checking email, seem tailor-made for someone with more power, autonomy, or money than me.

Tech Shabbat

One technique I recommend is taking a tech shabbat. According to Tiffany Shlain, author of the book *24/6*, a tech shabbat means going screen-free for a full twenty-four hours once a week. During that time, you socialize, play, create, rest, cook, and generally use the time however you'd like—just without the twitchy fingers and the mindless scrolling. I like it because it's straightforward. It doesn't require constant self-monitoring, which is cognitively taxing. There is only one decision to make: What day will you go screen-free?

My partner and I decided to give it a go. At the end of our experiment, we marveled at how easy it had been to ditch our phones. We made it through a playground visit, a lunch date, holiday shopping, and other errands with only minor inconveniences, and with ample generosity of spirit. When my husband arrived late to pick my son and me up from the playground, I wasn't resentful or annoyed. I figured he was doing his best. I had to let go and trust that he would be there soon, because I couldn't reach him.

Not having our phones also gave us a surprising burst of energy. Isaac sprang into action vacuuming the car (long overdue). I tackled a donation pile I'd been meaning to organize for weeks. Were it not for the tech shabbat, we both admitted, we likely would have disappeared into our phones during that time.

Doing this on a weekly basis turned out to be too ambitious for us— two parents with a toddler and a feisty rescue dog, with all our weekend playdates and visits with abuelos and tías—but it's something we'll likely do at least a few times a year. (Once a quarter seems more like our speed.)

Take a Mini-Break from Your Phone

If you can't unplug for a full day because of work or other responsibilities, start small and work your way up. Even a few hours of screen-free time can set you on a path to less compulsive tech habits, less worrying, and more relaxation.

Start by putting your phone away right now. Try to read the rest of this chapter without it by your side or in your view. When you've finished, check in to see how you feel. You may have some anxiety at first, but chances are you'll feel more liberated and relaxed once you've committed to it.

Continue to build up this muscle over time, gradually spending a longer period away from your phone. Challenge yourself to spend a few hours a day or more without your phone. You might even keep a log of your progress, which can motivate you to keep going.

Try a Tech Shabbat

You don't have to be religious (or even Jewish) to try a tech shabbat. It's really about reconnecting with what's most meaningful to you and choosing to prioritize this over meaningless device time.

To take your own tech shabbat, follow these instructions:

○ **Choose a time.** Following Shlain's lead, we powered devices down from Friday night to Saturday night. (We choose 5 p.m. as our start and end time.) Non-workdays are recommended, for obvious reasons.

○ **Let loved ones know,** and make sure you have at least a few emergency contacts memorized or written down, just in case.

○ **Plan ahead, or don't.** Improvise your meals or print out recipes in advance. Create a detailed itinerary for the day—or skip the planning altogether.

- **Celebrate.** Today is a special break from your routine. Find small ways to mark the occasion, whether that's hosting a dinner party to kick things off, bringing home a nice bottle of wine or bouquet of flowers, or simply sharing highlights with friends and family at the day's end.

- **Keep it simple.** Shlain recommends using various accessories to ease into your device-free time, like a landline phone, a record player, a camera, board games, and magazines. If these items give you peace of mind or will make the day more fun, go for it. Otherwise, keep it simple. We skipped these and did just fine.

- **Invite others.** You can do a tech shabbat on your own, but it's infinitely more fun and easier if you do it with friends, roommates, or family. Having others join in also creates shared accountability, which helps you stick to it.

- **Invite abundance.** Your tech shabbat is not about sacrifice or deprivation, but intention and abundance. You are creating space in your day for the people and activities that are important to you. Use it to pursue the hobbies you love that always get pushed to the bottom of the list. Take it as an excuse to try something new. This is your time to explore and blossom.

Identity

Earlier we saw how societal pressures to be productive can make it difficult for just about anyone living in a capitalist society to slow down, pause, and rest. But for some of us, resting is not merely difficult, it is practically impossible. If you are part of a marginalized community— be it due to race, ethnicity, class, gender, sexuality, religion, disability, body size, or other differences from the "norm"—resting is likely to be both more out of reach and more urgent for you. This is especially true for those of us whose identities are at the intersection of multiple marginalized communities.

The experience of being on the margins often comes with discrimination, sexism, bigotry, homophobia, transphobia, ableism, and fatphobia, among (sadly many) others; navigating these challenges can be mentally, emotionally, and physically taxing. If you're part of a marginalized community, you suffer the consequences of being yourself—your wonderful, true self—because the system in place is designed for someone else.

Many communities are marginalized. Some examples are women, people of color, immigrants, LGBTQIA+ people, and disabled people, but this list is not exhaustive. Later, I'll dive deep into a few illustrative examples of marginalization; as you read on, think about how these challenges might apply to a marginalized community you or a loved one are part of.

If you are part of one of these groups, you will find familiar stories here, ones that I hope provide some comfort that you are not alone in your struggles. If you are one of the lucky ones who does not belong to a marginalized group, please don't skip ahead. Building an equitable society in which *everyone* has a right to rest is a burden we all share, and you are especially responsible if you are in a position of power.

Who Gets to Rest? Systemic Blockers to Rest

Whether due to race, gender, disability, class, or other forms of marginalization, certain groups undeniably have it tougher than others. Here are some of their stories.

The Trauma of Racism

Zee Clarke has all the trappings of a success story: She's Ivy League–educated, has worked at top companies in corporate America, and now runs her own thriving wellness business. But one day, as Clarke peruses the selection of tofu and tempeh in a supermarket in Northern California, no one sees any of that. All they see is that she's Black. After purchasing her groceries, she and a friend load up their car. And then a police car shows up.

"My heart rate shoots up. I have a terrible feeling in my gut, and I think to myself, 'Is this really happening?'" Clarke shared on Medium. The cashier has called the cops and accused her of stealing deli meats. Zhalisa Clarke is vegan, but that doesn't stop the police from searching her bags for the missing deli meats, meticulously cross-checking each item on her receipt. "It's 90 degrees and the ice is melting and my food is sitting out in the hot sun. I'm told not to touch anything. I'm told to sit down. After the item-by-item search, I ask permission to close the cooler. The $220 worth of groceries I had just purchased might go bad," she writes of the event.

It's moments like these that inspired Clarke to start her business, which specializes in breathwork and mindfulness training for people of color to help manage the day-to-day microaggressions and discrimination they experience. It also led to writing her book, *Black People Breathe.* When discrimination strikes, she takes a breath and releases a long exhale. She breathes through her belly. These techniques—invisible to the eye—help regulate her nervous system so she can get through these tough moments.

For people of color in the United States, Clarke's experience is unfortunately all too common. Every day, ordinary trips to the grocery store, playground, or office, or even a simple jog around the block, can quickly turn into moments of microaggression, racism, discrimination, and violence. Simple, human acts of living in the world can easily become psychologically damaging, or even deadly.

People who experience discrimination, racism, and prejudice face many negative health consequences. They are at increased risk of heart disease and diabetes. They experience high levels of stress, anxiety, PTSD, depression, avoidance, and emotional numbing. Discrimination and microaggressions can set off the body's alarm system, raising blood pressure and cortisol levels. These consequences hold true regardless of how high we climb the corporate ladder. According to Isabel Wilkerson, author of *Caste*, highly educated, wealthy people of color are not shielded from these effects. People of color at the top of their field, who are the first or one of the few from their background to "break the glass ceiling," face continuous stressors in this rarified space and experience a lower life expectancy as a result. For these reasons and more, rest is increasingly being understood not as a mere luxury, but as a racial and social justice issue.

One pioneer in this space is activist, artist, theologian, and founder of The Nap Ministry Tricia Hersey. Through her Instagram account, performance art, and book *Rest Is Resistance*, Hersey has become a leading voice on rest as a social justice cause. As Hersey's work shows, rest is not merely a means to recovering from discrimination and trauma, but a means of reclaiming sovereignty over one's body and challenging the status quo.

The Poverty Tax

Depending on how stable (and abundant) your income is, rest will be easier or harder to come by; rest, privilege, and class intersect every day. For example, gig workers, temps, seasonal workers, and service and hospitality workers piecing together a series of unstable jobs typically have little autonomy over their schedules. These workers must negotiate taking a day of rest not just with themselves, but also with their employers, and they may lack real leverage. Those in the care industry, such as teachers, childcare providers, and other caregivers, may have more stable work yet face similar challenges. Often filled by women and people of color, these roles are consistently societally undervalued and chronically underpaid. Workers in these roles are more likely to live farther afield from their workplaces and face longer (and stressful) commutes as a result. They may also share smaller living spaces with roommates and extended family—not necessarily the most restful environment. For individuals struggling to make ends meet, rest can be especially out of reach.

Research from economist Dr. Sendhil Mullainathan and psychologist Dr. Eldar Shafir suggests that financial scarcity is especially detrimental to our cognition. Scarcity leads to mental tunneling, or focusing on what is scarce (such as money) to the detriment of other areas. The result is a foggy brain, poor sleep, decision fatigue, lack of impulse control, and difficulty thinking clearly. In other words, poverty taxes the brain. The poor have fewer mental resources to work with in part because they are so preoccupied with making ends meet.

"If you want to understand the poor, imagine yourself with your mind elsewhere. You did not sleep much the night before. You find it hard to think clearly. Self-control feels like a challenge. You are distracted and easily perturbed. And this happens every day. On top of the other material challenges poverty brings, it also brings a mental one," Mullainathan and Shafir write in their book, *Scarcity*. Impoverished people have "lower effective capacity" than the rich "not because they are less capable, but rather because part of their mind is captured by scarcity."

Increasingly, rest has become a luxury item—one packaged in the form of pricey retreats, $200 weighted blankets, travel getaways, spa days, and other activities that are cost prohibitive for many people. Being able to take a sabbatical, retire early, or quit your job to recover from burnout, as I did, is only possible if you have financial privilege. Even taking a day off to catch up on sleep is a privilege—it requires having enough job stability that an ad-hoc day off won't disrupt your budget or job prospects. Many people don't have that flexibility. When you are working hard to make rent and get food on the table, rest becomes a luxury difficult to afford—financially and mentally.

Sexism's Claws

Like racism, sexism and gender discrimination against cis women, trans women, and transfeminine people surface in moments big and small every day. Having to carefully navigate how firmly or directly you express yourself, tending to the emotions of your colleagues, hiding or downplaying your ambitions lest you alienate your teammates, knowing that your male coworker is being paid more than you despite your experience, dealing with sexual harassment, receiving gendered feedback from your boss, and managing the implicit and explicit biases against women that exist in our workplaces—all of this takes a tremendous toll on women's health and well-being. Altogether, many women experience this as a perpetual state of stress. It is the cost of being a woman in the world, one that makes rest and recovery all the more crucial.

These biases exist not just in our workplaces, but in our homes and families too. Traditional gender roles create an imbalance in responsibilities. "I've been married for twenty-three years. My husband has never cooked a meal. As a woman, I feel the need to be the one to keep things together in the household, which is exhausting," Carla, a mother of two, told me.

In heterosexual couples, women often take on more of the "mental load" and housework than men do, yet more and more women are becoming breadwinners. "There's actually not that much of an expectation where you can exist on a one-salary household anymore. So now you need women's economic input, but you still have all the unpaid labor cards. Everything else is still on," Eve Rodsky, author of *Fair Play*, told me.

Though many women are desperate for "me time," it's usually the first thing cut from their busy schedules. Often, women with children combine their leisure time with childcare, a two-for-one approach that means they are efficient but never get real downtime. It is not uncommon to see a pair of mothers catching up while their children play—the efficiency of combining a playdate for the kids and social time for the parents is enticing. But with one eye still on the kids, mothers may find it hard to fully decompress. Conversation, which can be its own stress release, tends to center on the children too. A more restful approach might be to hire a babysitter or have a family member watch the kids and have an adults-only catch up instead.

Many women are accustomed to putting others' needs before their own, but this makes finding peace, ease, calm, and abundance difficult.

Changing the System

If you are a member of one of these, or any other, marginalized groups—and especially if you are a member of more than one of these groups—resting may not just *feel* more out of reach for you, but actually *be* more out of reach for you. You have the right to be angry at the lot you've been dealt. It isn't fair.

Although we may bear some personal responsibility for not getting the rest we need (which we will explore in chapter 3), we also need ambitious, systemic solutions to prevent the exhaustion and fatigue so many of us feel today, like having universal health care, universal daycare, paid family leave, better sick leave policies, stronger rights for disabled people, experimental community housing design, and a universal basic income.

SYSTEMIC SOLUTIONS to EXPLORE

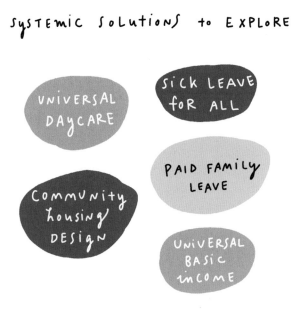

"There's a limit to how much individual strategies to achieve restoration can be sufficient when we have a society that doesn't offer paid leave or sick leave, and we have so many gig and occasional workers," says psychologist Dr. Darby Saxbe. "To me, rest means that when you have a baby, you have access to federal paid family leave, for example. That's what a society that values rest would look like. Whatever kind of individualized strategies that you can pursue, I think it's important to contextualize that they're deeply inadequate when you have a society that isn't really set up to permit people to achieve rest in any supported way."

To truly access rest, it takes individual change *and* societal change. We'll need activism, spiritual work, community work, raising awareness, fundraising—and plenty of rest to boost these efforts. This kind of systemic change is more complex than individual change, but it's equally necessary.

TAKE A MICRO-MOMENT OF REST

Humming Bee Breath

Zee Clarke, the author of *Black People Breathe*, suggests using humming bee breath (bhramari pranayama in Sanskrit) to manage your body's response to microaggressions. "Humming bee breath allows you to connect to your inner self and connect to our own inner vibration," she told me. "It calms you and relaxes the nervous system. It's also good for your immune system and reduces inflammation. It's very, very powerful." To reconnect with yourself and calm your nervous system, try this brief breathing exercise:

1. Close your ears with your thumbs and cover your eyes with your fingers.

2. Inhale through your nose.

3. On the exhale, hum for as long as possible.

4. Repeat for five to ten breaths.

At the end of your session, notice how you feel in your mind and body. Do you feel more settled and at ease?

Chapter 3

How We
Our

Get in Own Way

A s we learned in chapter 2, there are many external forces that can prevent us from getting the rest we need. Our societal infrastructure, including our class, gender, and race, play a large (some would argue, the biggest) role in determining just how much rest is within—or outside of—our reach. Cultural norms and expectations around work also play a role.

But as individuals, we bear some of the responsibility too. Despite our circumstances, we do have some agency in our personal relationship to rest—which means we can get in our own way if we aren't careful.

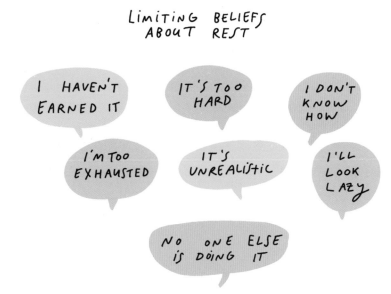

LIMITING BELIEFS ABOUT REST

I HAVEN'T EARNED IT

IT'S TOO HARD

I DON'T KNOW HOW

I'M TOO EXHAUSTED

IT'S UNREALISTIC

I'LL LOOK LAZY

NO ONE ELSE IS DOING IT

In this section, we'll look at how our upbringing, personality, and feelings and emotions can make it harder to rest, and what we can do about it. Let's start at the beginning.

Upbringing

Rani is a PR manager turned wellness practitioner. The oldest of seven, as a child Rani had a busy schedule during the week—between school, piano lessons, and other activities, her days were frequently full. But weekends were deliberately slow-paced. Her mother had a policy of letting the kids sleep in, and the house was often quiet till noon. Rani's days were intentionally unstructured, without agendas. "There was a freedom to rest," she told me. "Lots of sleeping and reading; never a push or pressure to be productive during the weekend."

Rani loved these slow weekends at home with her family, yet she couldn't help but feel tension—even resistance—from others in her life as she grew up. Friends shamed her for sleeping in instead of hitting the beach early on a Saturday. Coworkers did not see the value in setting healthy boundaries for rest, preferring to grind at all hours of the night.

"Seeing the norm as busy, you feel like you are the minority, and you begin to question that," Rani admitted.

Today, Rani is disciplined about prioritizing rest. She has learned exactly what works for her: Holistic practices like yoga, meditation, and walking in nature allow her to rest and recharge her mind, body, and soul. Even now, many of her friends don't understand why she left a plum corporate gig in PR to lead a slower-paced life. But she knows it is right for her.

Childhood Rest Begets Adult Rest

In my research on rest, I noticed early on a striking pattern: Our resting habits as adults are largely informed by our childhood. As children, we get many signals from the adult role models—parents, teachers, grandparents, or other caretakers—in our lives. If we grow up seeing our role models work late hours or during vacations, we may not think twice about doing the same. Alternatively, being raised in a family that values and regularly incorporates rest—be it in the form of play, sleep, exercise, or even spirituality—may make it easier for us to value and incorporate rest in our world as adults.

If you want to understand why you work, play, and rest the way that you do, take a look back at the environment you grew up in. It's likely you've held on to certain attitudes, beliefs, behaviors, and even coping mechanisms from childhood. Most of us build from what we experienced and what was modeled for us.

Uncover Your Personal Rest History

Grab a pen and paper and use the following prompts to conduct your rest history.

○ Think back to your closest childhood caretakers, whether those were your parents, grandparents, siblings, teachers, or other caregivers.

○ What was their relationship to rest like? What beliefs did they hold about rest? What examples did they set?

○ How did their behaviors affect your own rest and work behaviors as a child?

○ What attitudes, beliefs, and behaviors do you hold about rest today? How closely tied are these to your personal rest history?

○ Given what you have learned about your personal rest history, which attitudes, beliefs, and behaviors do you want to hold on to? Which do you want to let go of? Which might need adjusting?

SPHERES of REST INFLUENCE

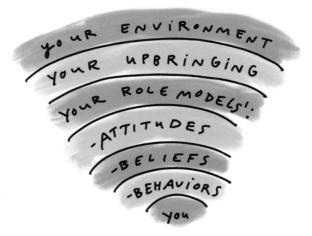

Don't worry if rest wasn't modeled for you in the way you aspire to rest today. Despite what you may have grown up with, you can still find a path to rest. In chapter 4 of this book, we'll learn techniques to help you do just that.

Personality

Our childhood experiences can explain much of how we relate to rest, but they are not the whole picture. I'm one of four girls, and though we all share the same set of parents, our responses to work and rest vary. We all work hard, but where I feel compelled to work first and play later, another sister is pulled to procrastinate. Two of us live by the to-do list; the other two are on their own timelines and don't mind doing things last minute or when the spirit moves them. These differences come in part because our parents were in a different stage of their work-rest lives for each of our childhoods (the span between the youngest and oldest is eleven years, so you can imagine the evolution). It's also because we're fundamentally different people, with unique personalities, coping mechanisms, and emotional experiences. It's a classic nature-nurture story.

However we grow up, our personalities are a part of what drives our actions and behavior. Certain personalities—and therefore behaviors— can make it both harder to prioritize rest and to rest effectively. Depending on your personality, resting may come more or less naturally to you than to others.

For example, if you are someone who holds very high standards for your work and believes each project must be perfect, that will likely affect your ability to switch out of work mode and into rest mode.

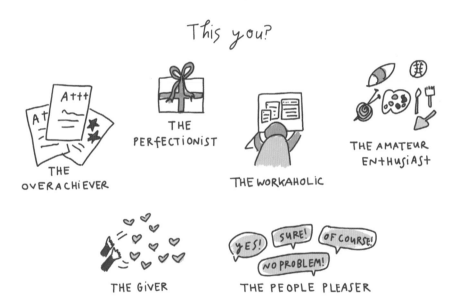

This you?

THE OVERACHIEVER

THE PERFECTIONIST

THE WORKAHOLIC

THE AMATEUR ENTHUSIAST

THE GIVER

THE PEOPLE PLEASER

Many of us fit into at least one of these groups—the overachiever, the perfectionist, the workaholic, the people pleaser, and so on—and we might not *want* to give up these traits. (As an overachiever myself, I look back on what I've accomplished and wouldn't trade it for a minute, even though I know I suffer the consequences of chronic stress.)

These traits are also difficult to change because they are so deeply ingrained in us. But it's important to bear in mind that they may negatively impact our personal quest for rest—or, at the very least, create some unique hurdles for us to overcome.

SELF-REFLECT: **Flip the Script**

Luckily, your particular personality alchemy doesn't preclude you from getting rest. You are not doomed to a life without rest if you're naturally high-strung or prone to workaholism. (Whew!) You just have to find the right outlet for these traits.

For example, if you're a natural go-getter, this doesn't mean you need to become less ambitious. (Easier said than done, anyway.) It just means you might explore other ways to express that trait. Instead of applying your hustle and drive exclusively to your career, where it is usually channeled, you might experiment with applying it to your social life, family, or community. Or, if you are a perfectionist at work, might you apply that attention to detail to designing a rest plan that works for you? And if you tend to be a "giver" who puts others' needs first, might you explore restful techniques you can do as a group to help others rest too?

Spend some time considering which of your personal qualities usually get in the way of rest. How might you leverage your unique personality as an asset to rest, rather than a hindrance or a liability?

The Five Rest Profiles

When you combine individual personality with societal circumstances and childhood experiences, you get a pretty clear picture of how you relate to rest as an adult. I call these *rest profiles*.

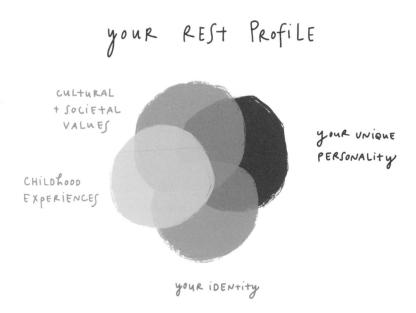

your REST Profile

CULTURAL + SOCIETAL VALUES

CHILDHOOD EXPERIENCES

your UNIQUE PERSONALITY

your IDENTITY

Here are five common rest profiles I've found in my research. As you read along, consider which feels most familiar to you. As with any set of profiles, it's likely that you will have elements of more than one. But one is probably a bit more "you" than others.

Intuitive Resters

Intuitive resters are in tune with their minds and bodies when it comes to rest. They recognize that when irritability, distractibility, and fatigue set in, it's best to slow down, not power through. They don't need to schedule reminders to rest because they've learned to recognize the signs in real time that they need a break.

Crucially, they are also in tune with what rest techniques work best for them. They may mix and match physical, mental, and emotional rest techniques or aim for more holistic solutions that address all three. Many Intuitive Resters incorporate rest directly into their routine—nightly shower rituals, daily walks, and pauses to appreciate nature make up some of the simple rest rituals they turn to. Intuitive Resters strongly believe in the restorative power of rest and take a diligent approach to integrating rest practices in their lives.

Functional Resters

Unlike Intuitive Resters, Functional Resters rest less by choice or enthusiasm than by necessity. Functional Resters may have chronic illnesses and require rest to stay healthy. Functional Resters may also work swing shifts or overnight shifts that require them to be sharp when the rest of us are sleeping. Whether due to health or profession, they do not have the luxury of regularly ignoring their need for rest—they *need* rest more than the average person in order to function without negative consequences.

Functional Resters rest due to their conditions, but begrudgingly so. Functional Resters are resigned resters. Because chronic illness, night-shift work, or other circumstances can get in the way of socializing, family gatherings, celebrations, and generally having fun,

Functional Resters may experience FOMO (the fear of missing out) and decide that it's occasionally worth ignoring rest so that they can see their grandchildren or attend that school play or family barbecue. However, these concessions are usually made sparingly, given their health consequences.

Gold-Star Resters

For Gold-Star Resters, rest comes only when they have completed their running to-do list for the day. It is a reward—a gold star—earned after other obligations are tended to. Unfortunately, such lists are often ever-growing, which means that for Gold-Star Resters, rest is often hard to come by. Although they know rest is necessary, and they may even recognize the signs that rest is needed, Gold-Star Resters frequently ignore this need in favor of being productive and getting more done. (It me.)

Given their (over-)achiever and task-driven nature, when they do rest, Gold-Star Resters are likely to schedule rest (for a later time, once other priorities are tended to), create rest reminders, and even set alarms to ensure rest is timeboxed around other activities. Because they are frequently exhausted by the time they allow themselves to rest, they often choose activities that seem restful but are not actually restorative (such as alcohol, television, and social media).

Unlike Functional Resters, when a Gold-Star Rester deprioritizes rest, they seldom face immediate negative consequences. Rest-resisting behaviors do, however, compound over time, often surreptitiously. Gold-Star Resters are prime candidates for suffering from chronic stress and burnout.

Anti-Resters

Like Gold-Star Resters, Anti-Resters frequently deprioritize rest in favor of other activities. Yet their motivation is different—rather than being driven by achievement and a desire to be productive, Anti-Resters can't sit still because they fear what this says about their character. They have internalized the message that "busy is best" and that idleness means they are "lazy." (This is also known as idleness aversion.)

"I grew up as a competitive athlete. You learn to be mentally tough. Just move on, keep going, don't think about your feelings," Erin, a single mom, says of her anti-rest mindset. Many Anti-Resters enthusiastically embrace "rise and grind" culture and may even perceive rest as a weakness. Whereas Gold-Star Resters want to rest but put it last on their list, Anti-Resters don't want to rest at all.

Unsurprisingly, many Anti-Resters also have trouble knowing exactly *how* to rest. The lines between their hobbies, passions, and second jobs are blurry, making it hard for them to know when they are in play mode and when they are in work mode. This makes fully decompressing a challenge.

Deprived Resters

Members of this group have their hearts and minds in the right place, but the circumstances are all wrong for getting the rest they need. Deprived Resters simply cannot rest no matter how much they wish to prioritize it. Consider: parents of young children, gig workers, hourly shift workers, and others who are frequently not in control of their own schedules. Hormonal changes (such as in pregnancy, postpartum, perimenopause, and menopause), sleep apnea, physical and mental illness, and other clinical disorders can also prevent Deprived Resters from resting well. We are all Deprived Resters at some points in our lives, but some of us are perpetually stuck in this category.

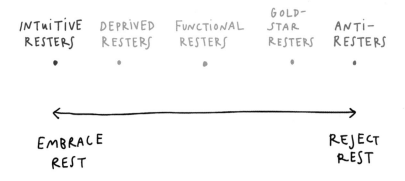

SELF-REFLECT: **What Kind of Rester Are You?**

After reading through the five rest profiles, which sounds most like you? Why do you think that is?

What kind of rester do you aspire to be? For most of us, there will likely be a gap between where we are today and where we want to be. Keep this in mind as you discover rest techniques in chapter 4 to transform your approach to rest.

Feelings and Emotions

Whether at home or at work, beneath the persistent drive to do more is a set of feelings and emotions that affect our rest attitudes and behaviors. These feelings influence how we make decisions and how we self-regulate when emotions and stress are high. On a good day, feelings like calm, anticipation, joy, and excitement come up when we think about rest. But often these feelings are tempered, mixed in with more negative feelings.

"It's okay to be excited about going to sleep and feel guilty about family at the same time. It's normal!" Swapna, a social worker, mother, and caretaker of her ill wife told me. Whether we experience feelings of guilt, anxiety, shame, or uncertainty around rest, the negative can coexist with the positive. We'll look at some of the thornier emotions that can emerge in response to rest now.

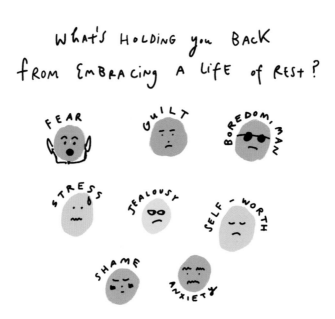

WhAT'S HoLDiNG you BAcK fROM EmBRAciNg A LifE of RESt?

FEAR GuILT BoREDOM, mAN STRESS JEALOUSY SELF-WORTH SHAME ANXIETY

Guilt

When Tanisha, a stay-at-home mom living with Crohn's disease, gets sick, she doesn't think about her own well-being—she worries about who she might be letting down. "Even though I'm violently ill, I feel guilty that I'm resting and not doing something for someone else. It feels selfish," she says.

Guilt arises when we think what we are doing is bad. Sometimes feeling guilty is warranted, such as when we know we've hurt other people. But many times it is a form of self-reproach: We judge and monitor our behavior and blame ourselves for failing to do (or be) what we believe is expected of us. If we think that resting may harm, offend, or disappoint others, we feel guilty and don't do it. Like Tanisha, many of us feel guilty about resting, even when it isn't warranted.

Guilt is a natural response, but it isn't always a helpful one. "The question I'm asked most often is 'How do I set boundaries without feeling guilty?'" writes Nedra Tawwab, a licensed therapist and the author of *Set Boundaries, Find Peace*. But according to Tawwab, "there is no such thing as guilt-free boundaries. Guilt is a part of this process." It's normal to feel guilty, but we shouldn't let that stop us from getting the rest we need. Guilt over rest is often a sign that we care deeply for others, but we also need to remember to care for ourselves.

Shame

Whereas guilt assumes we are a good person who has made a bad choice, shame suggests that our choices must make us a bad person. We may experience shame if we believe, as so many do, that resting is a personal shortcoming. Whether due to unspoken cultural pressures or interpersonal dynamics, we may feel that resting makes us weak or a bad person and be ashamed of our decision to take a break. This is especially true of Americans who have internalized the idea that work is a virtue, and who have confused self-worth with output. Yet resting is nothing to be ashamed of, and it has little to do with how good a person you are. On the contrary, to rest is to give yourself a chance at being the best version of yourself possible.

TAKE NOTE: **Friends and Family**

Family and social obligations are some of the leading causes of guilt and anxiety about getting rest. Certain relationships, especially those with a boss or parent, can trigger these feelings more readily.

Many of us have rich social and family lives that bring great joy and relief to our days. But it would be disingenuous to imply that friend-and-family time is all sunshine and roses. More often than we might like to admit, these responsibilities are in direct conflict with our desire to rest. Sometimes we are happy to partake, but other times we are just plain tired and in need of some "me time." Instead, we may feel obligated to keep the peace, go to restaurants we'd never choose on our own, or participate in vacations we'd rather not join in on—in short, to put others' needs before our own. Friend-and-family time can be fun and restorative—when we have a choice in when and how we partake.

Family relationships also come with responsibilities, whether you have children, siblings, an elderly or unwell parent, or a partner with mental health issues to take care of. It can be difficult to listen to our own needs and rest when we are taking care of others.

We all want to be there for the people we love, whether that's our chosen family or blood family. But like the airline safety messages say, it's important to remember to put our own oxygen mask on first. For most of us, that is easier said than done. In chapter 4, we will learn more about how to take small moments for yourself so that you can also be there for others.

you CAN LOVE your fAMiLy and
fRiENDS and StiLL fiND the tiME
with thEm StRESSfuL.

Stress, Worry, and Anxiety

To rest is to surrender, something many of us struggle with. Despite our desire to rest, we may have a hard time accepting it. Ironically, it's common to experience feelings of stress, anxiety, and worry when we think about resting. These feelings typically arise when we feel we *could* be doing something else, and indeed believe we *should* be doing something else—like caretaking or working—rather than resting. (This is also known as trade-off thinking, which we'll learn more about in chapter 5.) But if we are always wondering whether it's the right time to rest, it will be impossible to let go and relax. For those of us who believe rest is "earned" after accomplishing other tasks, feelings of stress, worry, and anxiety frequently keep rest at arm's length, since there is always something else we could be doing.

On top of our anxieties about rest, many of us also feel what Dr. Wendy Suzuki, neuroscientist and author of *Good Anxiety*, calls everyday anxiety—the kind of low-grade but chronic anxiety that has come to be accepted as a side effect of modern life. Seemingly minor stressors, like public speaking, running late to an appointment, or your first day at a new job, can trigger low-grade anxiety for many of us. So, too, can the fear that we are not doing enough or moving fast enough, or that we are missing out—the kind of worries easily triggered by an overflowing inbox or barrage of social media images.

When we experience stress and anxiety, our fight-or-flight system becomes activated to protect us against stressors and threats. Unfortunately, this system often responds with little nuance—whether a stressor is truly dangerous (a lion chasing after you), minor but overblown (a first day back at the office), or even imagined (imagining all the ways you might die in a car crash while safely driving). Anxiety can hold us in a persistent state of hypervigilance, stuck in a danger mode or worry mode even when it isn't necessary, making it difficult to relax.

Although it generally gets a bad rap, anxiety serves a real purpose: It is part of a natural stress response that tells us when change or action is needed. It is the kick in the pants we need to prepare for that presentation or leave early to get to our appointment on time. It is a sign that we care—about whether our children feel supported, whether our work is good enough, or whether we are spending enough time with our friends and family.

Regret

Unchecked, anxieties over whether to work or rest can easily morph into regret over how we've used our time. Instead of being happy we took the time to ourselves, we may begin to wish we'd taken care of the chores, played with the kids, called home, sent off one more work email, or handled whatever other responsibilities are haunting us. Uncertain about whether we are using our time well, we may struggle to commit to our decisions about rest, work, and play with confidence.

"Sometimes I think, 'I snuggled with my daughter today, but maybe I should have played with her in a more active way instead.' The only time I can rest without regret is when no one needs me," Erin, a single mother, told me.

Despite these feelings, it's likely that you're already doing the best you can, and that rest—as uncomfortable as it may feel at first—is just the right thing to do.

Follow Your Nose

Our sense of smell is uniquely linked to the hippocampus, where memory is processed and stored. According to Dr. Suzuki, scents that evoke "warm and fuzzy" memories can be grounding in moments of anxiety. We can also choose scents that are unrelated to an existing memory but create a sense of calm or joy. By doing this, we create positive associations between scent and feeling.

After you've finished reading this chapter, take a moment to do some olfactory exploring. This can include smelling essential oils, perfumes, flowers, herbs, spices, candles, incense, or even food. Before investing in any new scent products, raid your kitchen, which is chock-full of scents to choose from. Once you've found your calming, memory-inducing scent, keep it on hand for anxious moments.

Self-Criticism

We all have a voice inside our heads—and no, that doesn't make us crazy. Sometimes that voice is kind and compassionate, encouraging us to take a break, decompress, or try new things. Sometimes that voice is judgmental, bossy, and highly critical—the kind of voice that tells us we don't deserve rest, even when we do. This voice can be particularly vocal when feelings of worry, shame, and regret are involved. Unfortunately, when we engage in negative self-talk, we tend to focus on the bad and lose perspective of the bigger picture. We tend to believe we should have done better, known better, or tried harder. We get stuck in an unproductive cycle with ourselves—ruminating, worrying, and replaying a conversation, event, or decision in our head that we wish we'd handled differently. This critical voice tells us we should have worked harder, taken fewer breaks, or slept less to get the outcome we desire. It's hard to make space for rest when the most critical version of yourself has the mic.

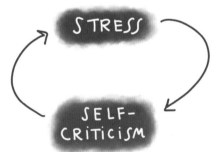

Research from Dr. Ethan Kross, a psychologist studying the science of introspection and how self-talk influences our emotions, shows that negative self-talk influences everything from our mood to our decision-making, reasoning, focus, creativity, and chronic stress. The more stressed we are, the more overwhelmed we feel and the more negative or persistent our self-talk can become. Over time, prolonged stress taxes the body and can lead to a decrease in appetite and sex drive and an increase in sleep disorders. The more self-critical we are, the more we push rest out of reach, physically and emotionally.

Luckily, there are many proven techniques for speaking to ourselves with self-compassion rather than self-criticism. In chapter 4, we'll look at these in more detail. For now, the next time you hear your inner voice judging or ruminating about whether you've worked hard enough or have earned the right to rest, ask yourself, "What would a friend say to me?"

Fear and Uncertainty

For many of us, resting feels a little bit like feeling around in the dark: We fumble, fail, and get lucky from time to time, but ultimately need a light to guide us through. Many of us simply don't know how to rest.

When we don't know how to do something, feelings of fear and uncertainty can set in. In response, we may distract ourselves with the familiar instead of trying something new. Fear can cause us to feel stuck in place.

Procrastination is fear by another name. When we procrastinate on a project, we do so in part because we are afraid to tackle it and afraid to fail. Rest can be similar: We may put it off because we don't know how we would fill the time when we're not working or caring for others.

Yet fear can also make us bold with adventure. We can channel our fear and uncertainty into experiments and exploration. If we are patient as we explore, we learn to keep trying until we get it right. Try to remember this as you explore rest practices and find what works for you.

Reactance

My nephew hates the idea of having a bedtime. He's a teenager, so he doesn't like being told what to do. As a result, he fiercely resists the idea of having a consistent bedtime, even though he knows he would benefit from it.

Adults do this too. You may know that exercise is good for you but refuse to lace up those running sneakers. You don't *want* to exercise—not if your partner is going to keep crowing about how you ought to do it.

Why do so many of us resist doing what we know is good for us? *Reactance* is the psychological term for why we chafe at others' advice or demands. If it feels like these demands are limiting our personal freedom, we tend to do the precise opposite. In other words, we take a strangely immature stance on something—the opposite of what's being recommended—just to preserve our personal sense of freedom and free will.

When we resist what we know is good for us, we have to stop and ask ourselves why. Just what are we afraid of losing control of? Can we find some personal agency in the matter? For example, setting a bedtime doesn't have to feel like a limitation if we reframe it as an opportunity to design how we end our day. We get to choose what note we end the day on, and how we end it. That leaves us happily in control and on a path to feeling well-rested—because *we* chose it.

SELF-REFLECT: **Feelings and Emotions about Rest**

Answer the following questions to unpack how your feelings and emotions influence your relationship to rest.

○ Which emotions stop you from developing good resting habits? How do they get in the way of resting? For example, perhaps you feel guilty about taking time for yourself if it means putting family second.

○ Where do these feelings stem from? Notice whether these are internally motivated or externally driven.

○ Are these emotions worth holding on to? Think about times in the past you've let a feeling or emotion stop you from resting, and what the results were.

○ The next time this emotion comes up, what is one thing you could do to manage it and still get the rest you need? For example, you might try a catchphrase ("Taking care of myself doesn't make me a bad parent; it makes me a responsible one") or remind yourself of what the research says ("Stress contagion in house-holds is real; I will de-stress to prevent making my family more stressed and miserable").

Chapter 4

How   to

Rest

TECHNIQUES TO ENERGIZE
AND CALM YOUR MIND,
BODY, AND SPIRIT

I n this chapter, we'll explore tried-and-true techniques for how to get the rest you need. Perhaps you have ideas for where to begin but are in search of inspiration and know-how to put those ideas into practice. Maybe, if what you tried before has failed you in the past, you are ready for a fresh start. Wherever your jumping-off point is, this section has something for you.

Whether your need for rest is mental, physical, or spiritual, you'll find a trove of recommendations to pick and choose from. All the rest techniques here are stress busters, anxiety relievers, calm inducers, and mood boosters—bound to help you relax, recharge, and feel restored.

These techniques are also what we call positive or adaptive coping mechanisms, which help you to positively approach a stressor or challenge. They are both effective and good for you—intended to help you recharge in a healthy way and to thoughtfully integrate more rest and rejuvenation into your life.

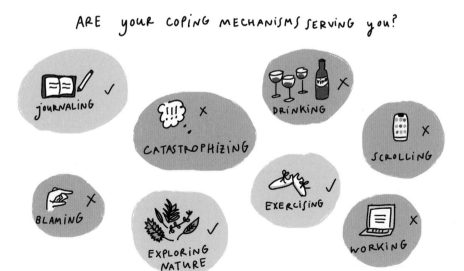

ARE your COPING MECHANISMS SERVING you?

JOURNALING ✓

CATASTROPHIZING ✗

DRINKING ✗

SCROLLING ✗

BLAMING ✗

EXPLORING NATURE ✓

EXERCISING ✓

WORKING ✗

Rest Your Mind

Like so many of us, it's hard for me to quiet my thoughts. Sometimes, I am on the verge of a panic attack and have to talk myself out of it. Other times, I'm ruminating on a situation I wish I'd handled differently or composing an email in my head instead of paying attention to my surroundings.

Many of us struggle with what Buddhists call "monkey minds": overactive minds that are restless, distractible, and unfocused. These active thought patterns—a mix of mundanities, negative self-talk, and self-doubt—can make it particularly challenging to let go and relax. Thinking can quickly turn into overthinking: questioning, spiraling, ruminating, and getting stuck in unhelpful, and unrelaxing, thought patterns. Rather than delight, inspire, or relax us, overthinking generally leaves us feeling stressed and mentally fatigued. It's hard to rest when we are caught up in our concerns, whether those are existential (like whether or not to have children, given global warming) or trivial (like whether to book your nail appointment for 11 a.m. or 1 p.m.—you maximizer, you).

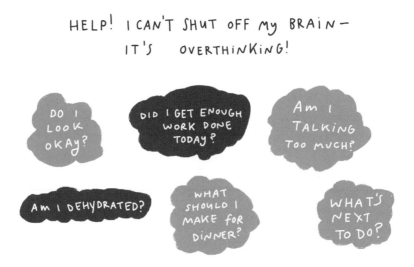

In the pages to come, we'll learn how to turn down the noise in our heads, make space for serenity, and begin to find peace of mind.

Worry Not

Some of the biggest causes of our mental unrest are the worries, stresses, and anxieties we carry with us every day. Worry can be triggered by a toxic workplace, a difficult relationship, a cross-country move, finances, child-rearing, health concerns, crowds, elevators, small parking lots, driving at night, deadlines, pandemics, climate change, small and hot spaces—just about anything, really (fabulous, I know). Even the most laid-back among us worry from time to time.

Unfortunately, worrying is at odds with our quest for rest. Usually, worrying involves ruminating on a past event or worrying about the future (also known as pre-worrying); when we are worrying, there's very little space to simply *be* and enjoy a quiet, restful moment.

Luckily, there are a few tried-and-true techniques you can employ to quiet your inner worrywart or nervous Nellie and be cool as a cucumber instead.

Practice Distancing

One of the best ways to manage your worry is to practice distancing. Psychological distancing is the process of zooming out from our worry to see the bigger picture. When we broaden our perspective, we are able to see the situation more clearly and less emotionally. We tend to find more solutions to our problems and, equally important, more acceptance of them.

DISTANCING HELPS US SEE
THE BIGGER PICTURE

STEWING

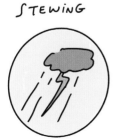

DISTANCING

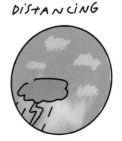

Psychological distancing is particularly helpful for ending cyclical chatter or rumination, and it is far more effective than distracting ourselves from our thoughts with social media or email, which doesn't get to the underlying wound.

One simple way to practice distancing is to speak to ourselves in the second person ("you") rather than the first person ("I," "me," "my"). Research from psychologist Dr. Ethan Kross shows that using the second person helps us create distance, improve our reasoning and problem-solving, and more effectively manage our stress. Calling yourself by your name ("Ximena, you've got this") is one of the fastest ways to regulate your emotions from fight-or-flight to being back in a balanced, calm, compassionate, and relaxed state of mind.

Another way to practice distancing is to think about what you might say to a friend in a similar situation. We often do not speak to ourselves with the same care, grace, and affection we offer to our friends and family. Imagining someone you love—or even yourself as a child—in your situation can help you to see your circumstances and your own behavior differently. This helps us go beyond what we feel are our own personal failings and helps us to be more self-compassionate. Gaining perspective in this way helps us to change our tone from one of judgment ("You're a failure") to one of understanding ("You did the best you could given the circumstances"). This usually leaves us feeling lighter, more focused, and calmer.

For similar reasons, journaling is another effective way to practice distancing—like the techniques mentioned above, journaling allows us to change the narrative of what we've experienced, so we begin to see things differently. We'll learn more about this technique later in this chapter.

SELF-REFLECT: **Identify Your Worry Pattern**

○   Take a moment to list everything that makes you worry. What topics, people, activities, or environments give you most cause for concern?

○   Look for patterns in your list. How frequently do you worry about these things? What kinds of worries come up the most? For example, do you tend to worry more about people, projects, places, or activities? Which worries cause the largest stress response? The smallest?

○   What coping mechanisms do you tend to use to manage each worry? Are they maladaptive (like using alcohol or drugs, blaming others for your problems, workaholism or staying busy to avoid your feelings, and putting others' needs above your own), or adaptive (like naming and talking about your feelings, self-reflecting, seeking support, engaging in hobbies, and saying affirmations)? Are they effective?

○   Where might you need a new coping mechanism? Think about which coping mechanisms pair best with the kinds of worries you encounter most often or most intensely. Keep this in mind as you explore the rest techniques throughout this book to find what works best for you—and your worries.

Explore Color to Stop Rumination

Sometimes, our thoughts begin to spiral. If you find yourself ruminating, getting lost in your worry, and having difficulty focusing, try this simple but important trick from Meredith Arthur, mental health advocate and author of *Get Out of My Head*, to quiet your mind and find calm.

Look around and name the colors you see. Say each color aloud: ocean blue, seafoam green, fire-engine red, and so on. The more vivid the description, the better. Allow yourself to be transported back to the here and now as you notice each color. Describing and naming colors in this way helps you get out of the mental loop and into the present. Use color as a gateway to feeling grounded—away from our internal chatter and toward peace and ease.

Focus

Growing up in New York, I went to museums often. As a child, I'd wander the galleries with a little sketchbook in my hand. When I found something intriguing, I'd stop and sit with it for five, ten, fifteen minutes. As I looked, I sketched—paintings, drawings, sculptures, found objects, conceptual art. The more I stayed with each artwork, the more I started to make meaning of them. I lingered on the impossibly thick paint strokes, the perfect sheen of a sculpture, and the puzzle of a found object. I began to see that what appeared to be a single color from a distance was, upon closer inspection, actually achieved through half a dozen colors. (I also loved hunting for the artist's signature—a sort of game I played to keep me engaged with every piece.) This process could be calming or energizing, depending on the kind of art. Years later, I still find it meditative and enthralling.

Most of us walk through life with scattered attention and distracted minds, pulled by technology, to-do lists, and multitasking. Yet with focus, we can tame the stress and overwhelm that usually accompanies these activities. Whether we aim our attention on art, nature, or even a good meal, we can find calm simply by focusing. Giving something our undivided attention, if we know where to focus it, can be pleasantly absorbing and mentally restorative. Here are some suggestions for how to direct your attention to find peace of mind.

Find Flow

As a child, I didn't have the words to describe why my museum experiences were so restorative; it wasn't until adulthood that I understood that I was finding "flow" in sketching. Flow, as defined by psychologist Dr. Mihaly Csikszentmihalyi, is the experience of becoming happily lost in an activity. When we are in flow, we are completely absorbed in the task at hand. These tasks are usually ones people enjoy and find meaning in, and which are both challenging and doable. We can find flow in writing, painting, ceramics, music, and other creative pursuits, along with sports and even work we find meaningful. When we are in flow, our ego—the inner critic and inner monologue—tends to quiet. The key to finding flow is focusing on one thing at a time; there is no room for flow if we are multitasking or distracted.

To practice finding flow and quiet your mind, carve out thirty to sixty minutes of uninterrupted time—time you won't be interrupted by others, or yourself—and find a meaningful activity to get lost in. The right activity will be challenging yet achievable. (Too easy an activity can leave us bored, while too difficult an activity can leave us stressed.) I call these "stretch" activities because they require us to gently stretch our limits, without being impossible to do. (Drawing was achievable, but also challenging for me.) What might you find flow and relaxation in?

Practice Soft Focus

When we are not in flow, paying attention can feel forced. (Just think how hard it can be to stay attentive during a webinar, meeting, or even family dinner sometimes.) It takes concerted effort to voluntarily direct our attention on something and keep it there.

Thankfully, looking at nature gives us a break. "Soft focus" is an open, soft, informal monitoring of the environment, and it is easily engaged when we focus on the natural environment. Because the brain is familiar with (and, indeed, evolved to recognize) organic shapes and forms, it is engaged but not overtaxed. This kind of focus is involuntary and effortless. According to attention restoration theory, paying attention to nature doesn't drain our brain resources and is actually restorative. When practicing soft focus, we may experience awe, empathy, and calm.

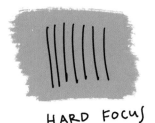

HARD FOCUS

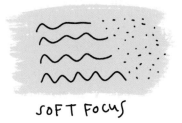

SOFT FOCUS

Before you shoot off another email, take a moment to simply look at the leaves of a nearby tree fluttering in the wind. If you are lucky enough to live or work by the water, stop to enjoy the rhythm of the waves for a minute. When you are feeling stressed or simply want a mood boost, pause to take in the sunset or watch the clouds drift by. These small moments can all elicit positive feelings of awe. Later, we'll learn more about how being in nature—not just looking at it— can further activate our rest response.

Observe the World Around You

Whether you are in nature or a city, a museum or a supermarket, observing your surroundings can be a helpful way to find peace of mind. Take a moment now to carefully notice the world around you. Notice the sounds, textures, movement, and interplay of objects and people nearby. Focus on a specific moment, scene, or place and see what you can discover. What happens when you use all five senses to observe the world around you? What new things do you see and feel?

Mind-Wandering

Some days, it will be harder to find focus and flow than others. When we are distracted or bored, it can be difficult to pay attention. Rather than concentrate on what's in front of us, our minds often begin to wander. Mind-wandering can happen during low-pressure activities, like washing the dishes, and high-pressure ones, too, like an important team meeting at work, a difficult conversation with a loved one, or a challenging interview.

When our mind wanders, the brain gets a break from paying attention. That allows other ideas to surface. This explains why we daydream, make mental lists, readily flit from one topic to another, enjoy word-association games, and have our best ideas in the shower. It's also why we might get stuck making to-do lists when we ought to be sleeping, or why we are unable to focus on that boring Zoom call despite our best efforts.

Though at times frustrating, the brain evolved this way for a reason. Mind-wandering is a feature of the default mode network, the part of the brain that is active during rest states. This mode is responsible for our ability to be introspective, empathic, and creative. It is part of what makes us social creatures, able to imagine what it's like to be someone else, and able to connect and commune with others. It is also why we share stories and updates about ourselves. When we feel we are not in control of our thoughts, the default mode is likely activated.

When our attention wanders, it can be tempting to try to snap it back to reality. But sometimes the most restorative approach is to simply let go and relinquish control of our attention. Here's how.

Embrace Boredom

For many of us, before we can even identify the feeling of boredom, we have reflexively grabbed our phones or other devices in an effort to rid ourselves of it. There is a slight lull in the conversation, so we fill it with something shiny (a tweet, an article, an email). Ditto for passing the time in line at the post office, waiting for the pizza delivery to arrive, or even while in the bathroom. We use multitasking as similar armor against boredom; when we are not engaged enough to stick with something 100 percent, we simply add something else to the mix. Unfortunately, in our efforts to rid ourselves of boredom, we tend to turn to non-restful activities, like mindless scrolling, list making, or busywork.

Discomfort and boredom are signs that our brain wants to do what it evolved to do—wander. Boredom can be uncomfortable, yet if we continue to comfort ourselves with distraction, we deprive ourselves of a chance at relaxation. Boredom is also beneficial for creativity and problem-solving. Rather than resist boredom when we are experiencing discomfort and are prone to distractibility, we can embrace it instead. We can protect ourselves from adding more hurry into our lives by welcoming boredom instead of swatting it away. To reap the benefits of boredom, we have to learn to withstand the discomfort it brings.

You can start by resetting your expectations of what you think will be boring. What might happen if you welcome possible boredom instead of arming yourself against it? Try people watching at the grocery store instead of texting. Notice something new on the drive you take to work every day. Take a walk and leave your phone at home. We can turn small, ordinary moments into playful, energizing ones with a shift in intention and attention.

Honor Tiny Transition Time

Often, it's the small moments that can make us feel busiest if we aren't careful. Moving from the living room to the kitchen, or while waiting at a stoplight, we may reflexively check our email or cue up a podcast. Instead of busying ourselves during these tiny transitions, we can honor these small moments by doing nothing and letting our minds wander. Look for moments of transition in your daily life to see where you can create more space to give your brain a break. Honoring these tiny transitions as phone-free moments is a bite-size way of encouraging your mind to wander.

Try Creative Waiting

Rob Walker, author of *The Art of Noticing* and the popular newsletter of the same name, recommends showing up early to take in your surroundings. He calls this creative waiting.

"One way to give yourself a break is to show up early. I'm always early, because I hate to be late, but I started treating that extra time differently," he told me. "Instead of being irritated at it being 'wasted,' I treated it as a tiny vacation—a moment to people watch, examine a space, or even close my eyes and zone out. This way if I make it a point to arrive fifteen minutes early, I get a fifteen-minute break.

And if my date is late, well, more free time for me!"

The next time you have an appointment, try getting there fifteen minutes early. You can also try this when faced with a delay in your day (while waiting in line at the grocery store or post office, or for your turn at the doctor's office, for instance). Use this time to check in with yourself and how you are feeling, to take in your surroundings, or to simply enjoy a moment unhurried. After your session, reflect on how your creative waiting went. What did you learn about your surroundings? How do you feel now?

Daydream

As a kid, you may have been told to get your head out of the clouds. If you were a daydreamer in school, your teachers likely tried to snap you out of it. While it's true that daydreaming in the middle of class or a high-priority meeting might not win you favor among your teachers, bosses, and colleagues, in the right situation, daydreaming can provide the perfect mental break. While riding the bus to work or driving to pick your kiddo up from daycare, let your mind wander and invent worlds old and new. At the beach or park, dare to get lost in your own thoughts and stories. You can even daydream in bed (yes, the erotic kind of daydream—everyone deserves a little pleasure). In search of inspiration? Swing by your local library and peruse the stacks. Surrounding yourself with others' stories can inspire your own.

Swap Meditation for Meditative Activities

Like many, I've dabbled in meditation. And like many, I've struggled to really get the hang of it. Many of us aspire to meditate as a way to calm our restless minds but find it difficult to master and commit to.

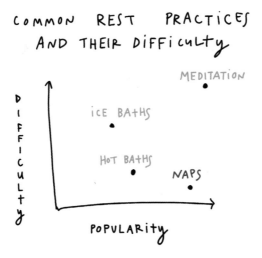

COMMON REST PRACTICES AND THEIR DIFFICULTY

Meditative activities, such as meditative walking, tea meditation, savoring a meal, bird-watching, and candle meditation allow a quieting of the mind that may be more accessible than traditional meditation. They work by giving you something to focus on during your practice, be it the scenery, the warmth of your tea, the spices in your food, a bird overhead, or the brilliant flame of a burning wick. When a thought arises, you can focus your attention back on what's in front of you.

Simple, repetitive activities may also be helpful, such as knitting, embroidery, fishing, drawing, pottery making, puzzling, gardening, or even washing the dishes—without a podcast, TV show, or other distraction in the background. These are engrossing activities that allow the mind to wander.

MEDITATIVE ACTIVITIES

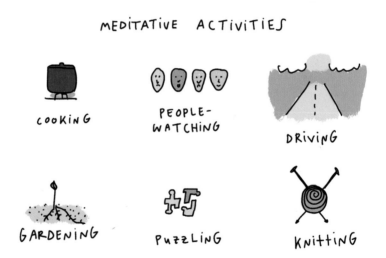

COOKING

PEOPLE-
WATCHING

DRIVING

GARDENING

PuzzLiNG

KNITTING

Finally, activities that allow us to engage in procedural thinking—which is repetitive, how-to thinking that involves know-how, such as juggling, bookbinding, or even following a recipe—also help to quiet our minds.

At first, focusing on what needs to happen next in the procedure offers instant relief from rumination. Over time, as these steps eventually become second nature, these procedural activities serve as a springboard for mind-wandering.

SELF-REFLECT: **What Activities Are Meditative to You?**

To find the right meditative activities for you, try the following:

○ Make a list of activities you find meditative—activities during which you either "stop" thinking, find flow, or peacefully allow your mind to wander. My list includes things like knitting, drawing, walking, petting the dog, and driving.

○ Look at your list with discerning eyes. Which of those activities is easily accessible (not costly, requires little setup, and easy to incorporate into your daily routine) to you?

○ What's your meditative activity? How might it fit into your world?

When I look at my list, I am forced to be honest: I have not knitted in twenty years, and I'm not likely to get started now without incurring a setup cost. I love drawing but it can also be a little stressful now that I do it for a living. For me, driving to pick my son up from school is the ticket—it's a route I'm familiar with, and so long as I don't listen to a podcast, I can let my mind wander freely as I drive. For someone who generally hates driving, I've come to find the ritual strangely relaxing.

Try Doodling

You don't have to be an expert artist to take advantage of this simple mind-wandering trick. Grab a piece of paper and a pencil (or a pen, if you dare) and follow your hand as it makes shapes, lines, figures, and forms as if on its own. Your doodles can be fancy and picturesque, or simple and unrecognizable (you can toss them in the recycling bin as soon as you're done, if you'd like). The goal is to create space on the page for your mind to unload its burdens and simply wander. Doodling is simply mind-wandering or daydreaming on paper.

When I doodle, my mind surprises me with the feelings, thoughts, and memories that surface. I'm always intrigued by what comes up—each thought is a tiny snippet into my state of mind.

As you doodle, allow your mind to wander as it pleases. After a few minutes of doodling, notice how you feel. What ideas and thoughts came to mind unprompted? What feelings and emotions might need tending to? What did you learn about yourself?

Ride the Wave

If you feel a pang of boredom or an urge to give up on your meditative activity, or whenever you find yourself absentmindedly unlocking your phone, starting to binge-watch another episode, or seeking other distractions, give yourself fifteen minutes before giving in and trying to make those feelings of boredom and discomfort go away. Riding the wave, also referred to as surfing the urge, is the practice of noticing our discomfort and boredom and pausing before we respond to it. Specifically, we wait fifteen minutes and *then* decide if we are going to "give in" to the urge. Usually once those fifteen minutes have passed, so has the craving to rid ourselves of discomfort and boredom. A simple pause may be exactly what you need.

Curate

Although many of us think of space and setting as a mere backdrop to life's daily mundanities, psychologists and urban planners know that physical spaces affect our psychology and well-being. Certain environments are intuitively calming to us, while others drive up our stress levels. We take cues from our physical worlds all the time.

This is good news for aspiring resters—it means that we can design our environment in support of rest, if we know how. One of the easiest ways to cue rest from our environment is to curate our space. We can create a sacred setting to help us calm our anxieties and access peace, calm, and even joy.

Designing for Rest

Bringing a personal touch to a cold office environment might seem like a frivolity, but it can actually help you relax. Studies show that adding personal items in impersonal settings like offices can help relieve stress.

Color is an especially useful tool for improving your mood and inviting relaxation. Although you might prefer a muted palette, monochromatic grays, beiges, and whites tend to be unstimulating and can lead to restlessness and difficulty concentrating. On the other hand, bright, colorful spaces leave us more alert and boost our energy. Blues and greens are particularly restful; they help relieve stress and anxiety. A playfully organized room can bring a spark of joy or delight to our days (no wonder color-coded bookshelves are so popular).

To decorate for rest, think about the colors and objects that make you feel most relaxed. Consider painting your wall (if you are permitted to do so) or bringing in colorful accessories (blankets, picture frames, plants) to liven up your space and combat fatigue. Leafy, green plants are another way to quickly spruce things up—they help reduce stress and boost energy and concentration. Try bringing in a treasured knickknack or special photo to make you feel more relaxed and at home.

Listen

Whether it's music or rhythmic ocean waves, many sounds can provide us with opportunities to relax and help us calm our mind. From the sound of hair dryers and washing machines (a favorite among newborns and even some adults) to the pitter-patter of rainfall, sound can be a pathway into relaxation. Cinematic, nostalgic, poetic, lively and energizing or grounding and stabilizing—the right sound can transport us away from our worries to another time and place. Here are a few tunes to explore to activate your rest response.

Mindful Listening

I have no idea how much time has passed. I am lying still on my bed with an eye pillow on my face. Headphones in, I can hear cymbals shimmer and crash. Then come the singing bowls and a number of instruments I can't identify. The sounds, whatever they are, seem to move through me, no longer something I am listening to, but something I am a part of. For reasons I can't articulate, a scene begins to materialize in my mind's eye: I picture myself looking regal in all-white knight's armor, making my way through an emerald-green forest. An entire cinematic world unfurls itself before me and sweeps me away. So begins my first sound bath.

After my session, I am slightly disoriented, but satisfied—not unlike the feeling of waking up from a good nap. Immersing myself in the sound has distorted my sense of time, just like a dream would. How long was I lost in the sound? I can't tell, but I feel, intuitively, that I'd accessed something of depth. I was but a mere passenger on a journey through time, sound, and a fictional world of my own invention.

"Sound possesses a unique temporal nature. It sets the stage for us to enter liminal states, where time seems to elude us even as we're still completely in the present," Lavender Suarez, the sound-healing practitioner who conducted my session, writes in her book, *Transcendent Waves*. Spending time in that liminal space can be deeply restorative.

You don't need to go to a sound-bath session (although I quite enjoyed mine) to experience the benefits of sound's liminal states. We can use mindful listening for a similar effect without even leaving our homes. Mindful listening means giving our full attention to what we are hearing, and allowing ourselves to be transformed by it. Intentionally tuning in to the sounds of our surroundings allows us to transform a noise into a song, or a simple musical interlude into a moment of rest. "Not every sound is a song, but any sound can be part of a song, or built into one," Suarez says.

When we pay attention to the sounds around us, we change how we experience them. In these moments, it is not uncommon for time to feel as if it's slowed down—a rare gift in a world that seems to be forever accelerating. Here are some sounds to mindfully listen to and relax.

Nature Sounds

Studies show that nature sounds can relieve stress and help us to relax, stimulating our rest-and-digest system much like spending time in nature can. These sounds reduce our typically inward focus, pulling us out of our worrying cycles and toward the sounds of our environment. Birdsong, wind, and the sound of running water are particularly pleasing and effective. You can take a walk outside, visit a garden, or find a soundtrack with nature sounds to help you to relax.

Music

Music can be a powerful tool for evoking memories and moods, both energizing and calming. Our strongest music memories are formed in our teens and early twenties, which explains every generation's passionate nostalgia for their days of yore. You can boost your mood by choosing a song that takes you back to a happy time or place. Or calm your mind by listening to music that helps you relax—likely something slow-tempo and melodic, although your mileage may vary. What songs help you relax? Which help you to feel energized?

Silence

Silence can be its own sonic experience, if we pause long enough to pay attention. Silence helps us to concentrate, process information, and remember things. Silence has also long been an ingredient in traditions of spirituality, meditation, prayer, and contemplation. It is a chance to get lost in our thoughts or connect to a greater purpose.

Many of us crave silence but also find ourselves discomfited by it. "If I could just have a moment of quiet!" we think to ourselves amid the noise of family or city life. But a curious thing happens when we finally do get these moments of auditory respite—we fill them with sound.

I noticed this myself when I took a writer's retreat to work on this book. Though I had a decent office setup at home, home was filled with distraction and noise—my barking dog, my husband on work calls, and our toddler running, jumping, singing, and playing in the house. These were wonderful sounds of life, but not exactly conducive to getting a manuscript in on time. So as I neared my first deadline, in lieu of an official writer's residency, I stayed in a tiny home for two nights. The place was blissfully quiet—perfect for getting writing done. But during writing breaks—while cooking and eating meals, getting up in the morning, preparing for bed at night—without thinking about it, I did everything I could to break the silence. I instinctively turned on NPR in the mornings and my favorite podcasts at night. I listened to music at mealtimes. Although a part of me craved the quiet, I was having a hard time tolerating it.

When I finally realized what I was doing, I stopped. I felt myself twitch for my podcast app to turn on a chat show, but I rode it out. I let the quiet in—and realized it wasn't so quiet after all: I had been masking the roar of the wind outside, the footsteps of a crow landing on the tin roof of the tiny house. I felt more a part of my surroundings, more connected to them. Without all that noise, I grew reflective. I had blocked out my thoughts with other sonic inputs, but now I could hear them. They meandered on their own, not unpleasantly.

It's not unusual in this day and age to find silence uncomfortable. But it can also provide some sonic breathing room for us to just *be*. One simple way to create small moments of quiet is to power down devices from time to time. Whether it's taking a walk without calling home to kill time, driving without a talk show in the background, or simply doing the dishes to nothing more than the sound of water gushing, look for small activities throughout your day to try in silence.

TAKE NOTE: **ASMR**

ASMR, or autonomous sensory meridian response, is a (largely anecdotally reported) phenomenon. Those who identify with feeling ASMR report experiencing a pleasant, tingling, calming sensation in response to certain audio-visual triggers, like the sounds of whispering, hair-brushing, and sorting trading cards. Although there has been little clinical research conducted on ASMR, millions watch "ASMR videos" meant to help them relax, de-stress, and even sleep better. For those who enjoy it, it can provide relaxation. Like listening to nature or music, ASMR encourages a kind of mindful listening that can be comforting.

Create a Sonic Sanctuary

Sonic sanctuaries are dedicated spaces where we can relax and feel inspired or creative. Filling them with peaceful sounds helps us to de-stress, improve our concentration and memory, and sleep better.

To design your own sonic sanctuary, find a cozy corner where you can be comfortable and inspired. Set up your spot with whatever physical comforts you need, such as candles, pillows, blankets, and photos that give you warm fuzzies. To keep things affordable, work with what you've got at home. Make a playlist, or perhaps a few—some relaxing, others engaging—for your sanctuary. You can rely on tunes you know and love or look for meditative music, singing bowls, or even Gregorian chants. Power up an ambience video conjuring a rainy day in a coffee shop, a cozy, snowy day by the fire, or a summer afternoon in the garden. When you're feeling depleted, take a moment in your sonic sanctuary to recharge.

If you're like me and live in an urban setting where space is limited, think of how you can use your surroundings to extend your home and create a sonic sanctuary outside of it. For some, a garden filled with birdsong can provide relief and inspiration. For others, a humming neighborhood coffee shop can do the trick. Even a blank page can offer a kind of silence and place for self-reflection. (Showers are great too.) What sounds and spaces feel most welcoming and restful to you? How might you design a sacred space around these sounds, at home and outside of it?

Rest Your Body

Kalalea's hands are impossibly hot. I am facedown on a massage table, fully clothed, with a sheet on top of me. I feel the heat from her palms as she presses one hand against my right calf and another against my lower back. She moves gently but purposefully, delicately yet firmly placing her hands on my body. Where she goes, the heat goes. *How is it possible to have hands this hot?* I wonder.

"That's the energy," Kalalea tells me later. I've just completed my first reiki session in an attempt to regain my stamina after a month of illness. It's been nearly six weeks since I've slept through the night without a coughing fit or stuffy nose, and it's dispiriting to be sick all the time, not to mention exhausting. A friend swore by reiki to help her feel restored, which brought me to Kalalea.

Reiki is a Japanese healing tradition based on the belief that the body can heal itself. In a reiki session, practitioners use precise, gentle hand movements above or on the body to relax and soften the muscle. This allows the reiki, or universal life energy that each of us carries within and around us, to flow through the body unobstructed and promote healing. (If the idea of an energy field sounds too out-there for you, just think about how easily you can pick up on someone's "energy" when they are stressed or in a bad mood.)

As with many traditional Eastern medicines, Western studies have yet to yield consistent evidence of reiki's efficacy. But for reiki adherents, it's the science that's not there yet. Many people swear by reiki for pain relief, stress, anxiety, and sleep issues, and many institutions prescribe reiki as a complementary treatment for patients.

After our session, I tell Kalalea that I felt pain along the right side of my body as she worked: My right wrist, IT band, and knee were all tender and achy. I even had a little bit of a headache on the right side. I wonder if that's normal. Could it be the result of poor posture? Maybe one leg is shorter than the other? (More common than it sounds!)

"Most people carry tension on one side," Kalalea assures me. "It is some-times tied to hand dominance," she says, and I nod in agreement—I am right-handed, after all. "The right side of the body is also the more mas-culine side. If anything has to get done, that's the right side," she adds. This is the part of the body associated with doing rather than being. The side responsible for taking charge and taking action.

"So the right side is my productive side," I say, laughing to myself.

Of course it hurt. Back then, all I ever did was *do*. My body wasn't used to relaxing.

Thanks to the mind-body connection, we know that stress, anxiety, and our mental well-being can manifest physically—through knots in our stomach, GI issues, tension headaches, and even panic attacks. Likewise, physical challenges can also affect our mental health; anyone who's had to recover from a physical setback knows how emotional and mentally exhausting the process can be. In this section, we'll look at the importance of getting the body the rest it needs. We'll learn how we can promote energy when all we feel is fatigue, how to access calm when our body is in fight-or-flight mode, and how to take care of our bodies in order to take care of ourselves.

Move

When I think about physical rest, I think of spas, sleep, maybe even a stretch or two. (Mostly, I think of lying down.) So you can imagine my surprise (and, truthfully, my dismay) when, during the course of my research, a handful of die-hard exercise enthusiasts in my life kept *insisting* that exercise could be restful. They waxed on about runner's high and the satisfaction of breaking a personal record on a bike ride. But how could breaking a sweat possibly help me rest? It was the least relaxing thing I could imagine.

At first, I ignored their suggestions. I stuck to my sound baths and breathwork and got through the first six months of my research in supine position. Until one day, I lamented to my husband that I once again felt listless despite getting a good night's sleep, and he said, with a look in his eyes I have come to know as a mix of gloating and admonishment, "You realize there's a very popular, research-backed solution to this, right?"

I covered my head with a blanket. "Don't say it," I groaned.

He cheerfully ignored me. "You're going to have to exercise."

We all know that exercise is good for us. It helps keep us agile, both mentally and physically, in old age. It enhances creativity and executive functioning. The right kind of exercise can even quiet the part of the brain responsible for planning, analyzing, and critiquing—the mental noise that makes it difficult for us to relax. Although I personally favored a kind of passive rest—a calming way to gently relax and refill my cup—I had to admit that taking a more active approach had its benefits. It was time to explore active rest and find invigorating ways to boost my energy.

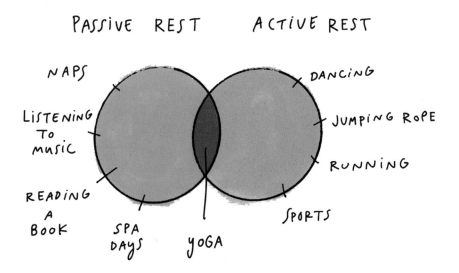

PASSIVE REST   ACTIVE REST

NAPS

LISTENING TO MUSIC

READING A BOOK

SPA DAYS

YOGA

DANCING

JUMPING ROPE

RUNNING

SPORTS

There are many different forms of exercise, at least one of which will be right for you. (If, like me, you are allergic to exercise, try reframing it as "movement" instead.) Maybe you crave high-intensity workouts like CrossFit or slow-paced ones like qigong. Perhaps you prefer solo ventures (and sweating in private), or maybe you enjoy the social benefits of more communal ones. You may like to keep it simple (no special equipment required), or try the latest gear and technical fabrics. As you consider the kind of movement that will work for you, remember to look for something fun, convenient, and accessible to help you stick with it over time.

Just about any kind of movement is good for us, but here are some options even many exercise-averse people, like me, can start with. They are especially gentle, which may be helpful for those who are exercising for the first time in a while, or for those with limited mobility. Of course, if you prefer something zestier, don't let me stop you.

Walking

What I love best about walking is that you can do it anywhere, anytime, in any weather. You can walk in a city center or out in the woods. You can get walking whether you're in great shape or taking your first step off the couch. You need no special equipment or gear. Walking is one of the most accessible forms of exercise.

Walking is also the perfect blend of physical and mental activity. When we walk (without our devices), the changing scenery helps us refresh our thinking. We allow our minds to wander: to ponder, problem-solve, and release whatever we're working on or holding on to. As we move through our environment, it's difficult to ruminate on one thing. Walking also aids in creativity, recall, mental health, mood, and autobiographical memory. And walking benefits us physically too: It is good for digestion and cognitive control, helps our organs repair from wear and tear, is good for the heart, and keeps us neurologically young.

Some of us can afford to take long, luxurious walks on our own, but many of us cannot; we have childcare, job responsibilities, and other realities of everyday life that get in the way. (There is a reason that most of the great thinker-walkers we know of are men—Henry David Thoreau and Walter Benjamin, to name a couple. I suspect they were free to write and walk because someone else—ahem, a lady—was responsible for everything else.)

Still, even the busiest among us can find ways to make walking work for us. Perhaps this means walking with your children or elders, even if that means going at a slower pace than you would on your own. (Take it as a welcome cue to slow down, if so.) Or perhaps this means taking a brisk urban stroll instead of a leisurely country walk. (Remember to look for blocks with extra greenery.) Maybe it's making an event of walking the dogs, rather than approaching it as a chore. Or perhaps it means simply extending an errand with a pedestrian detour or two. What would happen if you did an extra loop? Walked a few more blocks? Took a bit more time? Walk and find out.

Shaking and Dancing

If you've ever seen a dog have an anxious moment—barking at a mail carrier, villainous neighbor, or its Fido nemesis—you know it's usually a two-part process. First, the dog experiences stress. It may bark, jump, lick its lips, or growl when faced with its stressor. But then, once the moment has passed, it does something else: It shakes itself off from head to toe, releasing the stress with it. The full-body shake-off is like a giant reset button that clears the deck and takes our brave pup back to neutral. It's a quick and easy way to regulate stress levels and return to homeostasis.

Shaking our bodies can help us release stress too. Tanisha is a former dancer living with chronic illness; for her, dance—a more graceful way to get that full-body shake—is a crucial stress release. "As a child, dance was my escape from being sick, and an escape from some trauma that I had when I was younger. I always saw it as a safe space. When I dance, I don't think about what's going on in my life. It's almost like a pause, and I'm just at peace. I dance at home now, even just a few minutes a day, and that relaxes me," she told me.

You don't need to be a professional dancer to benefit from dancing your worries away. You might jump around, isolate and shake each individual part of your body, or simply do a full-body shake and get your wiggles out. Make your own moves at home: Play your favorite jams and bust a move for a minute. Go dancing with friends, or learn a new routine online. If time and budget allow, take a class to get moving (never have I had so much fun than when I took a West African dance class in college). Be the youngest person in your local Zumba class, or the oldest—who cares? Work your hips and the rest will follow.

Swimming

Midway through high school, I joined the swim team. What began as an excuse to spend more time with friends ended up being a key part of my adolescent rest routine. When I swam, all the noise in my head melted away. Sometimes, I counted strokes or laps back and forth, back and forth. Other times, I focused on the blue line at the bottom of the pool, tracing it with my eyes as I crossed the pool. It was quiet beneath the water. It was also blissfully repetitive—swim one lap, then another, then another.

Swimming is a proven mood booster, promotes relaxation, and is also helpful for anxiety. Bonnie Tsui, a former competitive swimmer and the author of *Why We Swim*, describes swimming as a "moving meditation." "The body is engaged in full physical movement, but the mind itself floats, untethered," she writes. Not only is swimming helpful for calming our anxious minds, but it can also provide physical relief: It stimulates mobility and circulation without pain, making it particularly good for injury recovery, pain relief, and arthritis.

If you have access to a pool or body of water, you might try swimming your worries and pains away. Check out your local public pool or gym for swim classes to get started. Once you're comfortable in the water, try lap swimming, which is likely to be the most meditative.

Yoga Nidra

Practicing yoga in any form is beneficial, but it's worth looking at your yoga practice to evaluate whether you have the right balance of active *and* passive forms of yoga.

If you've taken a yoga class before, you've likely spent some time in Savasana, or "corpse pose"—a pose in which you lie down on your back, relax, and let go of any tension. In many conventional yoga classes, Savasana is comically short (thirty to sixty seconds after ninety minutes of flow yoga). We have only the briefest of respites before getting back to our busy lives.

Yoga nidra offers an extended Savasana. Usually, class begins with a few stretches, then quickly transitions to exploring a state of relaxation. This entails lying on your back, supported by a bolster beneath your knees, perhaps with an eye pillow on your face and a blanket covering your body. As the instructor guides you to become aware of each part of your body, you begin to drift off. You fall into a kind of systematic relaxation, where you shift from a state of normal awareness to a deeper state of consciousness. (EEGs, tests that monitor brain-wave activity, show that we enter a deep, non-REM state, despite remaining fully conscious, during yoga nidra.) It's not quite a nap, but you're not quite awake either: You're in a state of in-between (perhaps not unlike a sound bath). In this space, "all that's being asked of you is to let go of 'doing' and be guided by grace back to the source of who you really are," writes yoga nidra instructor and author Tracee Stanley.

What would happen if you let go of "doing," as Stanley says? I struggled with this during my first yoga nidra session, but in exchange for sticking with it, I was rewarded with a deep sense of relaxation and rejuvenation. To find out for yourself, consider exploring yoga nidra classes near you. If your local yoga studio does not offer yoga nidra or if it is cost prohibitive, there are many guided exercises and classes online (some free, some paid) to help you through your practice and reach relaxation. With practice, you will find that accessing this liminal space becomes easier. Over time, you may even find that you can access yogic sleep without a guide—or, in other words, that *you* are the perfect guide for accessing ease, calm, and relaxation.

Stretch It Out

Stretching is a quick and easy way to incorporate movement into your routine, no fancy equipment or gym membership required. No matter how busy you are, everyone has enough time to stretch.

Take a minute to stretch whatever feels good right now. Try a head, wrist, or ankle roll, shake your hands and feet out, or even try a walking lunge or two. Feel the stretch and connect your breath to the movement, breathing into each stretch as you go. Stretch both sides out for parity. When you've finished, notice how you feel. Are you energized by this quick dose of movement? Feeling grounded? The next time you take a stretching break, see if you can stretch longer or deeper. Do the same with your breath. Each time you stretch, check in with yourself after and notice how your mood and energy lift.

Touch

How does something as simple as touch heal our restless minds and battered bodies? Whether it's a bear hug, a back rub, cuddling, sex, or holding hands, physical touch comes with many benefits. When we are scared, a quick hand squeeze from a partner lets us know that we are okay. When we are activated, placing a hand over a friend's heartbeat and another over our own can bring us back to feeling regulated. When we are exhausted, a warm embrace lets us know that we can stop powering through.

Physical touch has been shown to reduce blood pressure, heart rate, and the stress hormone cortisol, while increasing the feel-good hormone oxytocin. Massage therapy is particularly beneficial: Studies show that massage helps reduce stress, increase relaxation, and improve our mood and our alertness. It can also help with symptoms of anxiety, especially when combined with other treatments. Touch is a pathway to relaxation. It makes us feel good.

Touch has social-emotional benefits too. Many of us bond through touch. We may feel more connected to others with a hug from a friend or a hand on a partner's knee, especially if our "love language" is touch. Physical intimacy can help us feel desired and express our desires to others. "Skin-to-skin," the practice of placing a newborn on their parents' bare skin just after childbirth, regulates heart rate and breathing, reduces cortisol levels, and aids in bonding between parent and child. Even petting a dog can be a positive bonding experience, and it reduces stress and increases well-being.

TOUCH TELLS ME...

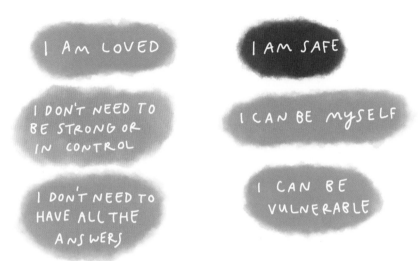

I AM LOVED

I AM SAFE

I DON'T NEED TO BE STRONG OR IN CONTROL

I CAN BE MYSELF

I DON'T NEED TO HAVE ALL THE ANSWERS

I CAN BE VULNERABLE

Although nothing beats a hug from someone you know and love, touching an object imbued with meaning can also bring relaxation in a pinch, be it a worry stone, a special ring or necklace handed down over generations, or simply a favorite sweater you always feel your best in.

Even our own touch can be beneficial. Many of us do this without thinking: We instinctively clasp our neck or touch our collarbone when we are nervous or feeling uncomfortable. We can self-soothe with a hand to our heart, a self-hug, or a touch to the cheek.

Touch and Be Touched

Not everyone finds physical touch calming (some of us even find it stressful). But if you're someone who finds it restful, there are a few things you can do to promote relaxation through touch.

Take a minute to hug a friend, kiss or cuddle a partner, or pet an animal to activate the stress-busting benefits of physical touch. If good company is sparse, try self-soothing by putting a hand to your heart. You might also touch something you find satisfying or calming—grab a stress ball, wrap yourself in a comforting blanket, skim a hand in a pond or bath, run your fingers across the bark of a tree, thumb a leaf or your favorite worry stone. After a moment, notice and appreciate how you feel. What feelings and emotions come up? How is your mood after a minute of touch?

Temperature

It was raining as we made our way up the mountain. My husband and I were on our way to a private thermal bath, where we would be meeting friends visiting from out of town. It was a special occasion (these were our first friends to visit in two years in a new city), so we'd taken the day off work to celebrate and reconnect. We would have ninety blissful minutes to rotate between an outdoor hot bath, a cold plunge, and a sauna while catching up on the last few years. But now the day was shaping up to be colder than expected. By the time we arrived, the rain had turned to snow. It was 45 degrees Fahrenheit (7 degrees Celsius), and a light breeze gave the air an extra chill.

After the obligatory flash shower (spa rules), I stepped out into the cold. The pool was only 3 feet (about 1 meter) away, but goose bumps quickly dotted my arms and legs. An involuntary howl escaped from my mouth, and I scrambled into the hot water. "Ahhhhhh," I half-yowled, half-sighed, releasing myself into the water. My muscles—wound tight to keep the cold out—began to relax and release tension. What had I been worrying about?

Hot, Hot Heat

Heat therapy—whether through a sauna, steam room, or hot bath—is a popular and effective relaxation technique. By increasing blood flow, heat helps relax our muscles to relieve stiffness, tension, and pain. Heat is not only useful for relieving aches and pains, but also for bringing us into a calm and cozy state.

You don't have to go to a sauna or thermal bath to tap into the power of heat. You can do this at home by wetting a towel and heating it up in the microwave, filling up a hot-water bottle, or simply taking a hot bath.

Just be careful not to go *too* hot—the temperature should be comfortably hot, not scalding. Also, be sure not to use heat on acute injuries, which can increase inflammation if applied too soon. (If the injury is fresh, it's usually best to go with an ice pack to reduce inflammation.)

Ice Cold

A hot bath can be relaxing, but nothing gets the blood pumping like a cold plunge. Cold water therapy can stimulate our fight-or-flight response, energizing us out of our fatigue. Cold water can help us snap out of it, whether "it" is rumination, fatigue, or depressive thoughts. It's a shock to our system that says, "Wake up! You're alive!" Especially when our mood and energy levels are low, cold water can be the kick in the pants we need to keep going. If you can feel how cold it is, congrats—you're still with us.

You can tap into the energizing effects of cold water at home by taking a quick cold shower, which can induce feelings of alertness thanks to the release of noradrenaline and cortisol. If jumping in a cold shower sounds like a nightmare (just me?), you might gently dip your face into a bowl of ice-cold water instead. This activates your parasympathetic response, helping you to relax.

As with all the techniques in this book, your mileage may vary. What's cold for me is hot for my husband, and what's unreasonably hot for me is totally comfortable for my son. Trust your body's response as you explore the thermal therapies that work best for you.

Sleep

Throughout my teens and twenties, I went through phases where I couldn't fall asleep. As soon as my head hit the pillow, my mind began to race: I couldn't stop thinking about all the things I needed to do (or wanted to do), or I would suddenly have a flash of insight that couldn't wait till tomorrow. It was a tug-of-war between sleep and my thoughts. Eventually, the longer I stayed awake in bed, the more likely it was that I'd find that my back or knee hurt, or that I was too hot or too cold, or both in a matter of minutes. Soon I'd be not only distracted mentally, but physically. I'd toss and turn and struggle to get comfortable. Even on miracle nights when I managed to fall asleep quickly and sleep eight or nine hours, it seemed to matter little the next day—I still woke up exhausted.

According to the CDC, roughly seventy million American adults are chronically sleep-deprived. Insomnia—the inability to sleep despite trying—is one of the most common sleep disorders. Sleep issues may be caused by illness, sleep apnea, chronic pain, mental illness, stress, grief, thyroid issues, genetics, environmental factors, lifestyle, and more.

Yet sleep is essential to our well-being. When we sleep, we strengthen our immune system, consolidate memories, and even uncover creative solutions to sticky problems (just ask the surrealists). Because sleep is such an essential part of our rest cycle (indeed, many people use the terms *sleep* and *rest* interchangeably), over the next few pages, we'll go deep into the benefits of slumber and how to access them.

Sleep Quantity vs. Sleep Quality

Sleep quantity refers to the number of hours of sleep you get per night. For adults, the gold standard is eight hours of sleep every night. Getting less than this, as most of us know, often impairs our cognitive and physical performance.

Sleep quality, on the other hand, is how good your sleep is—meaning how *efficient* your sleep is (how quickly you fall asleep at bedtime and following night wakings), how *interrupted* your sleep is (how frequently night wakings, particularly between 2 and 4 a.m., disrupt your sleep), and how *alert* your sleep leaves you (how energized or groggy you are during the day, without caffeine or a nap).

SIGNS of unHEALthy SLEEP

FALLING ASLEEP
TOO QUICKLY
(<5mins)

FALLING ASLEEP
TOO SLOWLY
(>30mins)

SLEEPING IN
ON WEEKENDS

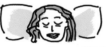

FRAgMENtAtioN
(FREQUENt NiGHT
WAKiNGs)

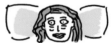

GRiNDiNG
TEETH

Sleeping Better

Most of us know the basics of good sleep: Keep your room at a cool 65 degrees Fahrenheit (18 degrees Celsius), don't bring screens into bed, and use your bed only for sex and sleep (not as a second office). Some of us have also tried blackout curtains, eye masks, earplugs, or even prescription sleep aids.

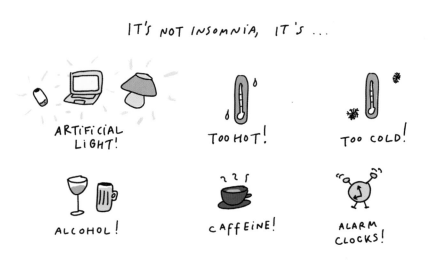

IT'S NOT INSOMNIA, IT'S ...

ARTiFiCiAL LiGHT!

TOO HOT!

TOO COLD!

ALCOHOL!

CAFFEINE!

ALARM CLOCKS!

If you're still struggling to fall asleep, stay asleep, or feel energized the next day, it is still possible to improve your sleep quality. Below are some recommendations for sleeping better.

Keep a Bedtime
Here's a small but important trick for improving your sleep: Keep a consistent bedtime, even on weekends. According to sleep researchers, this is the number-one thing you can do to improve your sleep quality.

Sticking to the same bedtime every night helps train your body to anticipate and welcome sleep, making it easier to fall asleep. Your brain learns to separate work time from rest time as a matter of routine, so there's no more mentally composing emails or planning a meeting agenda as soon as your head hits the pillow.

A good bedtime routine is consistent and includes some winding-down time to prepare for a good night's rest. In my case, the ritual begins an hour before bedtime: nothing fancy, just pj's, brushing my teeth, and reading a (physical!) book (usually fiction, but nothing too overstimulating). A few chapters in, I am ready to sleep. Sometimes I don't even make it to my 9:30 p.m. bedtime (yes, I am a grandma). Before, bedtime was haphazard—a thing that happened *to* me as much by chance as by necessity. Now it's something I *get* to do. I even look forward to bedtime now, rather than finding all sorts of clever ways (okay, mostly Netflix) to push it back. Years later, I still stick to these changes because they've helped so much. Keeping a bedtime has radically improved my daytime energy levels.

Eliminate (or at Least Reduce) Caffeine and Alcohol

Coffee and alcohol are some of the most popular vices in many of our regular routines. It's fun to feel uber-productive and focused after that first cup of the day, or loose and relaxed after a glass of vino at night. Unfortunately for us, these drinks come with unwelcome side effects on our sleep.

Caffeine negatively impacts our sleep long after its energy-boosting effects have worn off. Because of its half-life (roughly five to seven hours), half the caffeine of an afternoon coffee will still be working its way through your system ten to twelve hours later, when you are trying to sleep. Not surprisingly, this can disturb your sleep, both in terms of quality and quantity. As we grow older, it takes the body longer to clear itself of caffeine, making this a bigger hurdle over time.

Alcohol is also problematic for sleep. We may fall asleep quicker after drinking, but our REM sleep—important for consolidating memory and dreaming—is disrupted. Alcohol consumption usually leads to lighter sleep and more frequent waking throughout the night (including to pee or drink water), reducing our sleep quality overall.

Sleep researchers suggest cutting out caffeine and alcohol entirely for best results. As sleep researcher Dr. Matthew Walker puts it, "Nightly alcohol will disrupt your sleep, and the annoying advice of abstinence is the best, and most honest I can offer."

If complete abstinence feels out of reach, be judicious about when you consume what. Give yourself at least four hours between your last cocktail and your bedtime, and six hours between your last cup of coffee and your bed (or even more time, if you have trouble sleeping).

Avoid Energizing Activities Too Close to Bedtime

Eating, exercising, and napping can give us boosts of energy, which can be helpful early in the day but disruptive as we approach bedtime. Therefore, it pays to be strategic about when you engage in these stimulating activities. According to Dr. Daniel Jin Blum, sleep psychologist, it's best to eat your last meal of the day (ideally a smaller meal than breakfast and lunch) three hours or more before bedtime. Eating all your meals in an eight-to-twelve-hour span is best (be sure to eat your first meal of the day within an hour of waking up). When it comes to getting exercise, it's best to avoid exercising at night; aim for morning or afternoon workouts so that you can put that energy boost to good use. As for naps, these too should be carefully timed. For best results, don't let naps go past 3 p.m. Naps that run too late or too long can cause us to mistakenly push our bedtimes back further, subjecting us to shorter nightly sleep, leaving us tired during the day and . . . in need of a nap. You might also consider cutting naps out altogether if you struggle with insomnia—you want all the "sleep pressure" (which builds up over the course of the day) you can get to help ease you into dreamland.

TAKE NOTE: **A Note on Naps**

Sleep research shows that napping is a natural response to that afternoon slump we all hit (you know the one), and, *when combined with a good night's rest*, comes with benefits. As a routine event, it's good to nap—*if you're also sleeping at night*.

Napping *should*n't be a replacement for nightly sleep deprivation, which is how so many of us—college students pulling all-nighters to cram for exams, executives cutting sleep short to answer emails, or parents staying up all night with their newborn—use it today. Naps can help us recover from these events to a degree—when we are sleep-deprived, naps can help prevent us from nodding off into "microsleeps" or momentary brain lapses. But naps cannot salvage the brain from chronic sleep deprivation. A brain that is sleep-deprived struggles to make rational decisions, remember things, and provide emotional stability, which is why you're more likely to pick fights when you're tired. Naps can't help with that.

Of course, assuming you're getting enough sleep, it can be nice to indulge in a nap or two. If you nap, aim for ten to twenty minutes. According to Daniel Pink, psychologist and author of *When*, we should set a timer for twenty-five minutes in order to net approximately eighteen minutes of sleep. (It takes the average person about seven minutes to fall asleep.) As someone who sometimes struggles to fall asleep, trying to get something out of a twenty-five-minute nap stresses me out, but your mileage may vary.

Cut Caffeine

Many people love their caffeine habit, but it is not without negative consequences. Not only does it disrupt sleep, but it also affects energy levels throughout the day—and not in a good way. Anyone who has relied on coffee for a boost of energy knows that, eventually, the caffeine rush will wear off. Because caffeine only temporarily blocks out fatigue, when the energizing effects of caffeine fade, we feel worse than before. Caffeine withdrawal may be marked by headaches, fatigue, irritability, difficulty concentrating, and a decrease in motivation. The process of caffeine withdrawal starts while we are sleeping and peaks when we are waking up, which explains why so many coffee drinkers feel so miserable in the morning. Many of us get rid of this dreadful feeling by drinking another cup of coffee, not realizing that our caffeine habit is what's making us feel so bad in the first place. As journalist and coffee aficionado Michael Pollan puts it, "Daily, caffeine proposes itself as the optimal solution to the problem caffeine creates." The more you drink it, the worse you eventually feel, and the more you need it to feel better again.

What would happen if you eliminated your caffeine intake? Start by reducing your current dose to ease into the transition: If you're a two-cups-of-coffee-a-day kind of person, try making it through with one, or switching to decaf for the second. Cutting caffeine while sick can also help with this transition—when you're out of commission with a cold, no amount of caffeine can bring you back to life, so it's easy not to miss it. If complete abstinence feels out of reach, try a milder caffeine, like green tea, which has a gentler come-down. Because it contains less caffeine than your average cup of coffee, you can also drink multiple cups throughout the day without worrying about getting the jitters and overdoing it. Will there be some grumpy days as you battle caffeine withdrawal during this process? Yes. But it will be worth it in the end: Your energy level will be far smoother than the peaks and valleys that come with caffeine, and your sleep will be of better quality too.

De-Stress to Sleep Better

If you've ever gone through a phase where you needed more sleep than usual, chances are you were dealing with something stressful. Whether you're going through a major life event like moving across the country, managing a high-visibility project at work, or dealing with your toddler's transition from crib to bed, stressful experiences can impact how well you sleep. If your usual sleep schedule suddenly isn't yielding as much as it used to, stress may be getting in the way. "Life circumstances and stress can definitely affect the amount of sleep inertia, or grogginess, that you have during the day," sleep researcher Dr. Daniel Jin Blum told me. "During higher periods of stress, your body may need more sleep as well."

The bad news is that if you have a bad day, it's going to affect your sleep (thereby making the following day even tougher). You'll likely need more sleep. The good news is, if we can manage our daytime stress, we can prevent it from spilling over and ruining our sleep, which will ultimately make us less groggy the next day.

There are many ways to de-stress (the techniques in this book can help with that). Look for small ways to de-stress every day, such as deep breathing and visualization, repeating a calming phrase, getting exercise, socializing, or having some quiet alone time. Incorporate these stress-busting techniques into your regular routine, no matter how small they are. (You'll still feel the positive impact.) Pay attention to your stress levels and adjust your sleep and nap routines accordingly. ·

Keep Sleep Simple

Amid an array of potential sleep-aid products, there is a benefit to keeping things simple. "Usually I don't like my patients having a lot of *things*—like eye masks, earplugs, sound machines, humidifiers, weighted blankets, special bedding, and complete blackout shades. Not that they are not helpful—for some people they are a godsend. But on the other hand, the moment you add on another element, the reproducibility is going to be much lower for a nightly basis," Dr. Kin Yuen, a sleep researcher, told me. "If you need four factors to be completely perfect to produce one good night's sleep, it is not likely that's going to happen every single night." In other words, the more sleep accessories we employ, the higher we raise the bar on getting good-quality sleep. As you curate your sleep experience, be selective about what stays and what goes.

Manage Your Sleep Story

It's not only lifestyle changes that affect our sleep—our thoughts, emotions, and behaviors also play a role. In an interview, author and psychologist Dr. Adam Grant explains how the sleep stories we tell about ourselves can impact our actual sleep.

Grant suggests this is due to self-perception theory. "The basic idea is that a lot of times we learn who we are by observing what we do and say," he says. "And so if you hear yourself over and over again saying 'I'm an insomniac,' then pretty soon you start to internalize that as part of your identity, and then you feel all this anxiety every time you go to bed. And that just perpetuates the problem. Whereas if you stop saying that, what you've done is you've freed yourself from all the emotions that are associated with that identity."

Believing we have sleep troubles can become an unwelcome self-fulfilling prophecy. Calling ourselves insomniacs, or dreading bedtime because we are anxious about falling asleep, can make falling asleep that much harder. What sleep story are you telling yourself? What if you changed it?

Craft the Perfect Bedtime Routine—and Stick to It

To keep a consistent bedtime, you need the right routine. Follow these steps to find bedtime bliss.

○ **Set a bedtime.** For best results, work backward from the time you need to be up and give yourself eight hours of sleep to get there.

○ **Pick the right bedtime activity.** The key to keeping a consistent bedtime is to find some pleasure in your winding-down routine. Some people love a hot shower and aromatherapy. Others enjoy a crossword puzzle. Still others prefer to dim the lights, wave some incense, and light a candle. Whatever it is, indulge in the ritual of it—you want something that you'll miss when it's not there. Make sure your routine is enjoyable enough to beat out on other distractions, like social media, television, or other quick hits that can keep us up late with little payoff. (Those activities are also frequently used as a kind of "revenge bed-time procrastination"—a way to reclaim some time for ourselves after a busy day, but that usually just leave us more tired. For best results, your routine should be device-free.)

○ **Your new bedtime routine should feel like a little luxury or gift just for you, a kind of "me time."** If you find yourself pushing off your winding-down routine, you likely haven't cracked it yet.

○ **Keep going.** Consistency is key, especially when we are first forming a new habit. (More on that in chapter 5.) Do your best to hit that bedtime every day for the first week to gain some momentum. Some people find it helpful to give themselves a thirty-minute window of time rather than a specific bedtime (for example, 10 to 10:30 p.m. rather than 10 p.m. each night); others find that specificity to be helpful anchoring. Experiment to find what works for you, and keep going.

TAKE NOTE: **Check Your Cycle**

Women experience hormonal changes every month due to their menstrual cycle, which can affect their core temperature and sleep quality. Throughout the menstrual cycle, hormones rise and fall. Dropping estrogen levels can contribute to sleep disruptors like night sweats and hot flashes, while rising progesterone (the "relaxation hormone") and estrogen can cause sleepiness. Estrogen also affects the toning of the muscles around the airway, affecting breathing: During the first few days of the menstrual cycle, the airway tends to be slightly smaller compared to other days, which could create symptoms of insomnia. Such hormonal fluctuations occur throughout a woman's life—from menstruation to pregnancy, postpartum, perimenopause, and menopause. (Many forms of birth control, like IUDs and the pill, among others, can also disrupt our hormonal balance.) Unfortunately, as in other areas of women's health, much of the sleep literature skips over this.

"Nowadays we have to be our own detectives. I often tell women to keep a sleep log or use a sleep tracker so we can compare one day to the next," Dr. Yuen told me. She suggests paying attention to days where our sleep quality drops and tracking them alongside our menstrual cycle. Notice if you are spending more time at night kicking off covers to regulate your temperature, experiencing night sweats, or waking up more fatigued and having difficulty concentrating. "If the sleep quality for certain parts of the month are not as good as other days, then it does lead to some questioning: Could this be hormonally related?" If you suspect your hormones are affecting your sleep, it's best to talk to your doctor, who can refer you to a sleep specialist.

Try a Microsleep

A good night's sleep and a delicious nap can be a glorious thing, but sometimes we need a quick and easy way to recharge our batteries without all the bedding. When we intentionally close our eyes for a few seconds to a minute, we momentarily recharge our batteries.

Wherever you are, take a moment to close your eyes. Make yourself as comfortable as possible—lie down if you can, or simply lean back in your chair. Do not try to fall asleep; simply allow your eyes to take a rest from the stimuli of your surroundings. Allow thoughts to come and go as they please. Feel your breath lengthen. After a minute, open your eyes once more. Notice how you feel as you emerge from your micro-moment of rest. The next time you are feeling fatigued or overwhelmed and a nap or sleep is out of reach, simply close your eyes and breathe for a moment instead.

Rest Your Spirit

When we think of spirituality, many of us instantly think of organized religion. But you needn't be religious to be spiritual; your version of spirituality might include feeling moved by the sound of a song, taking a healing walk in nature, or experiencing harmony within a community.

Being spiritual simply means believing that we are part of something bigger than just us. It is finding solace in the idea that we are but a small part of the universe, doing our part to make a good life for ourselves and others. Being part of a community with others who share our values and beliefs can be comforting and grounding and help us feel less alone. Finding purpose and meaning in our lives can make us feel content, connected to something larger than ourselves. Believing in a higher being or universe can help us through grief and find healing. It can nourish our soul, emotions, sense of self, and purpose.

It's no surprise that to access these higher feelings, many religious communities and spiritual seekers espouse a regular day of rest—a sacred time to commune with themselves, others, and a higher being. It is a time to make space from the day-to-day routine—to step back from going through the motions and intentionally feed spiritual needs and connections instead. From the Jewish Sabbath to Christians' holy day of rest, this commitment to rest has existed for centuries. In many ways, rest and religion are intertwined.

Many spiritual practices have a calming effect. Some religious rituals, like praying the rosary, can be meditative and help with anxiety. Others, like the Quaker practice of sitting in silence, can help cultivate a sense of unity and connection. Practices like qigong, tai chi, and yoga, which have spiritual origins, can help us to feel more physically rejuvenated and at peace. For some, simply sitting in nature is a spiritual experience; taking in the sunset or the view from a mountaintop can promote relaxation and induce awe and a sense of being part of the natural world. People who enjoy tarot and astrology may find a similar spiritual connection in their quest for meaning and purpose. Even sports fans can be spiritual—they may follow their teams with religious fervor and experience a kind of ecstasy at a beautiful play or perfect performance. Whatever your spiritual practice or choice of god, you can find peace, joy, energy, and rest within it.

In this section, we'll explore the many ways to ease your spirit into moments of quiet, grace, self-compassion, and rejuvenation.

Nature

The connection between nature and our well-being has been well-documented. Spending time in nature improves our focus, attention, cognitive function, resiliency, and happiness. It reduces feelings of procrastination, distress, rumination, stress, chatter, and even the time it takes to recover from a surgery. After exposure to nature, time feels expansive, and we even seem to have greater impulse control (perhaps due to the sense of abundance nature often brings). As psychologist Dr. Ethan Kross puts it, "Green spaces seem to function like a great therapist, anti-aging elixir, and immune booster all in one."

One reason for this, biophilia, suggests that humans have a biological need to connect with nature because we are *of* nature; we're at ease in nature because we are of it. We hold an innate connection to nature and living things. We feel best when we are in "resource-rich" settings—lush with greenery, near a source of water—because they make us feel safe. Having evolved to thrive outdoors, we process nature easily (remember soft focus?) and more efficiently than urban settings. (Thankfully, research shows that even us city-dwellers can find relief—more on that in a moment.) The restful effects of nature are due in part to how easily we are absorbed by it. (This is the opposite of, for example, memorizing facts for an exam or talking points for a speech, which require effortful attention and can be draining.)

Nature's balm is one of the most effective ways to de-stress and access joy. When we take in the immensity of the Grand Canyon or an impeccable sunset, we may even experience awe. We feel more open, relaxed, and less time-pressured and impatient.

Here are some of nature's most powerful rest agents.

Sunlight

It doesn't take a clinical trial to know that sunlight is good for us—we intuitively know this to be true. Sunlight can boost our mood, alertness, and productivity. It can aid in how quickly we make progress at school or recover from a hospital stay. It also helps reduce blood pressure. There's a reason so many of us flock to the park at the first sign of spring or spend hours in the sun during the summer: It makes us feel good. You can even benefit from the sun when you are indoors. Simply follow the sun from room to room as it traverses your home throughout the day.

Trees

As kids, we learn that trees release oxygen and help us to breathe. What you might not know (or remember) is that they also release phytoncides, natural essential oils meant to protect trees from insects and fungi. These phytoncides protect the trees, but also protect me and you. Studies show phytoncides improve our immunity. They are anti-inflammatory, a sleep aid, and they have antidepressant properties. Most of us don't think of trees as anti-stress medicine, but that's exactly what they are.

In Japan, the health benefits of trees are taken very seriously. Shinrin-yoku, or forest bathing, is the act of spending mindful time among the trees, which is a national health project there (complete with designated "recreational rest forests"). What sets forest bathing apart from other activities among the trees is the intention to engage the five senses. Forest bathing can be as simple as finding a comfortable, pleasant spot beneath the trees (even a park will do), or it can be paired with other activities, like walking, yoga, meditation, breathwork, or foraging—so long as we stop occasionally to re-engage our senses in our immediate environment.

Japanese studies on forest bathing's benefits have shown its many positive effects on well-being, reducing stress, anxiety, anger, and depression; lowering blood pressure and blood sugar levels; and calming our fight-or-flight system. It has also been shown to boost immunity, cardiovascular health, mood, energy, concentration, and creativity. It helps to activate our parasympathetic (rest-and-digest) system and aids in sleep. In other words, it is a reliably restful technique.

Whether you commune with the trees by hiking in the forest, mountain biking, camping, walking in a park, or napping beneath a tree is up to you; the important thing is to make space for these calming trees in your life.

Plants

Like trees, plants are a boon for our well-being. They're also an easy way to bring a little bit of the forest—or the jungle, garden, desert, or meadow—to you. Plants not only offer many of the same benefits as trees, but can also whisk us away to another place or memory. Maybe you received a plant for a special anniversary or a job well done, or bought one back when you lived in a different city. Each plant marks a memory or a moment in time.

Tending to houseplants week over week, and if we are lucky, year over year, can be a spiritually fulfilling process. Here we are, nourishing this small, gentle plant, tending to it and caring for it in ways we want to be cared for too. (It is no wonder so many say that growing a plant is good practice for getting a dog, which is good practice for having a child.) In times of strife and through the occasional doldrums of everyday life, seeing signs of life—a bud, a flower, a fruit!—can be comforting. When we are personally responsible for this growth, the heart often swells.

Not everyone is a born gardener, but the beauty of houseplants is that there is something for everyone—from succulents and cactuses that require little watering to sensitive orchids that require just the right touch. Explore your local nursery and see what plants call to you. Ask which do well in direct sunlight, which can thrive in your shaded office, which can survive your forgetfulness and which cannot. Between their expertise and your instinctive pull toward a given set of plants, you're sure to find something you like—something to replenish your soul as your plant grows, bit by bit, toward you.

Fractal Patterns

As products of the natural world, we are naturally drawn to certain colors and patterns. We intuitively love saturated colors (blues and greens especially), repeated patterns, and organic shapes over linear ones. Fractals are particularly pleasing. These are organic shapes that look the same at any scale, no matter how big or small they are. For example, trees are full of fractal patterns: The smallest branch on a tree is similar to its largest branch in shape and form. These patterns are "self-similar," which means they repeat themselves within a single object or form, creating a sense of infinitude. Fractal patterns can be found in the leaves of a fern, the branches of a tree, flowers, clouds, foam, snowflakes, ice crystals, and even broccoli, among many other small natural wonders. Looking at fractal patterns is soothing in part because they are so easy for us to visually process. Luckily for us, fractals are everywhere, whether you live in a city or the countryside. In the park on a walk, or even at the grocery store, see what fractals you can find hidden in plain sight.

Negative Ions

Negative ions are invisible molecules in the air that are said to aid with mental clarity and boost our energy and sense of well-being. Most office spaces (and indoor spaces in general) have very low counts of negative ions. Instead, they are abundant outdoors, especially in sunlight and forests and near bodies of moving water. To get your dose of negative ions and boost your energy, open your windows and opt for a breeze instead of AC, give your dog an extra walk around the block, or take the longer route home if it means being outdoors and reaping the benefits for a little bit longer.

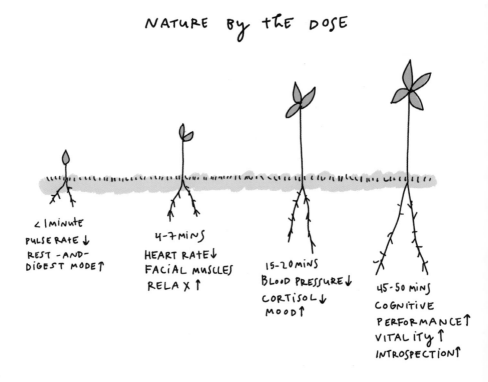

NATURE BY tHE DOSE

< 1 miNutE
PULSE RATE ↓
REST - AND -
DiGEST MODE ↑

4-7 miNS
HEART RATE ↓
FACiAL MUSCLES
RELAX ↑

15-20 miNS
BLOoD PRESSURE ↓
CORTiSOL ↓
MOOD ↑

45-50 miNS
COGNITiVE
PERFORMANCE ↑
VITALiTy ↑
INTROSPECTiON ↑

TAKE NOTE: **Nature and the City**

Regularly accessing nature is a proven stress reliever, yet today, most of us live in cities. Luckily, you don't need to move to the countryside or hightail it to the nearest forest or beach to access the restful benefits of nature—even city parks and gardens can be impactful. According to one study, spending just fifteen to forty-five minutes in a city park—"even one with pavement, crowds, and some street noise"—was enough to improve mood, vitality, and feelings of restoration. (In fact, research shows that just *looking* at photos or videos of green spaces can be good for our well-being.) No matter where you live, there's a patch of nature you can benefit from. Aim for five hours a month of green time, or just thirty minutes a day a few times a week.

Here are a few small ways to reap the benefits of nature and relax, even in an urban setting. Be sure to do these without your phone—using technology (texting, making phone calls, listening to podcasts) in nature diminishes its positive effects.

- Visit a park
- Look out a window toward trees
- Take a city stroll on the leafiest block you can find
- Look at pictures of nature
- Change your screen saver or device wallpaper to a nature shot
- Try a foresty essential oil (hinoki, Hokkaido momi, hiba)
- Pick up some indoor plants
- Do some window-box gardening
- Make like a cat and follow the sunlight in your office or apartment
- Listen to birdsong (on a recording, or in your own backyard)
- Take a lunch break outside
- Hunt for fractals in your surroundings
- Get your nature fill with a weekend trip outside the city

Beauty

My younger sister is a professional dancer, and whenever I watch her perform, a strange thing happens: I feel chills and get goosebumps, my throat tightens, and suddenly I am on the verge of crying. It is not just because she is my sister that I find myself so emotional (although that's part of it). It is also because I am in awe of what the human body can do. Whereas my own body is but a mere vessel—for work, toddler hugs, and getting from point A to point B—hers is a temple. She shows me what a body dedicated to art is capable of.

Sometimes we understand why something moves us, and sometimes we don't. Beauty's power works in mysterious ways. Like great art, beauty in all forms—natural, hand-crafted, or human-made—can be a healing salve, helping us to process emotions we might not have even known we were feeling. Making things beautiful, too, can lift our spirits and lighten our burdens—whether it's planting a garden, making pottery, or wearing something pretty.

Turning to art, music, and literature can be particularly grounding when we are going through a difficult time. Reading about grief can help us understand it, and watching comedy can remind us of the pleasures of joy. Following a character as they navigate feelings of loneliness or otherness can help us feel less alone in our own experiences. Listening to a melancholy song can surface a well of sorrow we didn't realize we were suppressing. Engaging with art can stir something inside us and help us make sense of it. When we immerse ourselves in a different world, be it one constructed with words, musical notes, or color, we can find an inner peace of our own.

Create a Beauty File

You can make space for beauty in your life in small ways every day. Start by making a list of things that inspire you or soothe your spirit. These may be songs, books, or works of art, or may include the names of your favorite flowers, trees, or grasses. Keep this file in a special place. When you feel the siren song of rest calling your name, choose an entry from your list to nourish your spirit. Crack the spine of your favorite book, hit play on your calming playlist, visit your favorite painting at the local museum, or venture out to see your favorite flower at a nearby garden.

Find Something Beautiful

Beauty needn't come packaged in a museum or gallery. Take a moment to examine your surroundings. Where might you find beauty? Look beyond the obvious. Beauty can be found in the color and shape of sunlight across your office floor, the smile of a child, the cozy texture of a perfect sweater on a cold day, the sound of the wind ruffling leaves outside your window. Find it and hold it in your eyes, hands, and mind for a minute, soaking it in. Notice what you are drawn to—what *you* find beautiful. Is it the textures? The sounds? The scents? No matter where you are, you can find beauty if you pause to look for it. The next time you are feeling low, remember to look for beauty.

Play

When was the last time you played? If you're like most of us, it's probably been a while. Many of us stop playing as we grow older: Who has time for a drawing class or bike ride when a deadline is looming? Who can curl up with a good book when the kids need their lunches packed and clothing washed? Responsibility, that hallmark of adulthood, regularly stops us from making time to de-stress and play.

Though we often associate play with children (it's also called "child's play" for a reason), it's just as essential for adults to play too. Play has been shown to boost creativity and productivity, increase optimism, aid in emotion-processing and decision-making, aid your immune system, reduce stress, help you build community, and restore your sense of self and purpose.

Whether it's getting silly to bring a little levity to an otherwise stressful situation, getting lost in a puzzle, or teaming up with friends for a round of trivia or pickup basketball, play is an essential stress reliever. We can try new things without fear of failure because the stakes are low. We can take our time because there is no need to rush through fun. We can explore, wonder, tinker, experiment, create, imagine, and tap into parts of ourselves long forgotten. Lost in play, we relax into ourselves. We enjoy the moment. We are present and content. We feel free and at ease.

In the following pages, we'll rediscover the activities that are personally regenerative to us—the ones that lift our spirits and nourish our souls—and remind ourselves of how to let loose and play.

Ways to Play

There are many different kinds of play. Free play includes telling stories, using your imagination, designing your own games, drawing, and other ways to play without rules. Structured play refers to playing board games, card games, sports, and any game with a healthy dose of rule-based competition. Skillful play includes cooking or other activities through which we can derive the pleasure of mastery. Meditative play may involve needlework, knitting, jogging, drawing, gardening, pottery making, fishing, and puzzles. There's even immersive play, such as reading fiction.

What ties these activities together is that each is something we can enjoy, get lost in, and feel rejuvenated from. (For this reason, common activities like scrolling social media or falling down a rabbit hole of Netflix episodes usually don't count as play; while we might enjoy these activities, they often leave us feeling worse afterward.) They're also activities worth undertaking for their own sake—for enjoyment, not solely as a means to profit, develop skills, or boost our LinkedIn profile. Unsurprisingly, we usually feel pretty good after a round of play (unless you are a sore loser).

Play is also highly personal—whereas mountain biking might be play for my husband, I'd rather curl up with a good book. Whether you prefer structured play or meditative play, the choice should, in fact, be yours— the most fulfilling kinds of plays are those that we *want to*, not *have to*, engage in. (This explains why so many corporate offsites fail to hit the mark on fun.) Only you get to decide what counts as fun.

There are many ways to incorporate more play into your life. Round up a group of friends for a rousing game of kickball or charades, or cozy up with a good book to transport you somewhere else. Invent new worlds of your own through writing, drawing, or even building blocks. Hike, dance, sing, play an instrument, bake a cake, knit a scarf, or put a puzzle together. Make art, browse a bookstore, or start a collection of treasured objects. Where you can find flow and fun, you can also find relaxation, contentment, and rest.

PLAY is...	PLAY is NOT...
PLEASURABLE	BORING
A GET-TO	A HAVE-TO
INTRINSICALLY MOTIVATED	EXTRINSICALLY MOTIVATED
A GIFT!	A CHORE

Find Your Play Zone

As adults, it can sometimes be hard to tap into a spirit of play—some of us are a little rusty. To find the kind of play that's right for you, think back to how you played as a child, or what play expert Dr. Stuart Brown calls your "play history." Answer the following questions, inspired by Brown's "play history" method, to help you uncover your personal play zone:

o **Make a list of your happiest moments and activities as a child.** When did you experience moments of unbridled joy? What made you happy? When did you get lost in flow? What were you doing? (If accessing your childhood is too painful, you can always pull from the recent past for inspiration.)

o **Look for patterns in your list.** Were these activities primarily mental or physical? Solitary or communal? Creative or logical? What qualities emerge?

o **What did those moments of play feel like?** For example, did you feel bold, nurtured, unique, or scared? Excited, in control, or curious? Try to get beneath the activity and connect with what it *felt* like to play.

o **What activities might help you tap into those feelings of play today?** Use your original childhood play activities as inspiration, but don't feel beholden to them. Your list might include those activities, new ones, or a mix. For example, if you were a bookworm as a child, reading would be an obvious form of play for you. But you might also enjoy browsing bookstores, joining a book club, or writing short stories.

○ **What hurdles might you face in your pursuit of play?** Hurdles can be physical (tender knees), financial (too expensive), logistical (time, equipment), or emotional (fear of failure or embarrassment). Although it's easiest to focus on logistical blockers, be sure to do some digging on emotional blockers too. It's amazing how often our own emotions prevent us from pursuing things we love.

○ **Start with an itsy-bitsy play plan.** Given your expected hurdles, what is a pared-down version of play that can work for you? For example, maybe you'd love to take a life drawing class but aren't able to given your busy schedule. Could your mini-play plan be to borrow a book on illustration from the library and spend a few minutes reading and drawing from it before bedtime instead? Or, if you are afraid to get started, what's one small step you can take today?

○ **Once you've found a play activity you're excited about, set aside time this week to try it.** If you find yourself dreading your planned play activity, punting on it, or just not having fun with it, don't force it. Go back to your list and try something else instead.

TAKE NOTE: **Paid Play**

In an age of constant pressure to monetize our hobbies and find a job that loves us back and pays us well, does commodifying a hobby or working at a job you love count as play?

In my experience, if you are paid for (or are trying to get paid for) a hobby or activity, it's no longer pure play. Money turns something we love *for the sake of it* into something we are *obliged* to do—for our bosses and our bank accounts. More often than not, what the commodification of hobbies offers is financial gain, not relaxation. It is nearly impossible to keep a pure relationship to play when a paycheck is involved, even if it is not the initial motivation behind our pursuits. (This tends to hold true even if you don't "need" the money, since money is also a marker of achievement.)

Some of us will eventually, even accidentally, make money from play. If what was once pure play is now a paid gig, find something else to fill your cup.

Travel

Travel can awaken our senses, desires, hopes, and dreams. It can connect us with moving, soulful experiences—be it through beauty, good food, a sense of adventure, or an inarticulable, deep connection to a place or its people. Travel can sharpen our observation skills, pique our curiosity, and inspire us to try new things. It can energize us like no cup of coffee ever could, or it can relax and nourish our soul like a long day on a lazy river. It can be replenishing and stimulating and calming all at once.

Many of us feel free and untethered while traveling away from home—the physical displacement leads to a psychological one, where we are more willing to try new things than before. Being in a new environment is like having the slate wiped clean: If we are timid at home, we can be bold abroad. If we are workaholics, we can be gluttons of rest. If we are bored and fatigued, we can become curious and energized—simply by being in a new environment and having an open mind. Each place we visit teaches us something new about ourselves—about what we find joy in, what energizes and inspires us, and what soothes us. I look back on my own travel experiences, and it's like I was a different person—an easygoing, carefree, unhurried version of myself.

Although some of us will be eager to cash in our airline miles and get out of Dodge, accessing the joyful openness that comes with traveling to new places can also happen closer to home. We can be a tourist in our own city or try a new nearby campground and adventure locally. We can read books and magazines about far-flung places. We can learn about other cultures through museum exhibitions, television, foreign films, and documentaries, finding wonder and relaxation through these vicarious experiences.

Of course, while the occasional travel adventure can provide a welcome change in perspective and help reset how we think about rest, to fully reap the benefits of these revelations, we need to cultivate an ongoing practice of rest that sustains us beyond our travels. We'll learn how to do this in chapter 5.

Heal

No one gets through life without a few emotional scrapes, but some wounds cut deeper than others. Whether we carry big-*T* Trauma (such as divorce or abuse), little-*t* trauma (such as the smaller conflicts and stressors and big feelings we navigate every day), or collective trauma (such as pandemics and wildfires), we all have reasons to want to heal.

Carrying trauma within us can take a physical, emotional, and mental toll. It can be difficult for us to get through the day, much less get some rest, when we are plagued by intense and painful memories or fears or are unable to move past a prior event. If we are stuck on a painful wound, we may find it difficult to relax.

Healing helps us move forward—to keep living, loving, feeling, breathing, giving, caring, and doing. When our confidence or sense of self is shaken, healing grounds us once more. When we feel weak, healing helps us feel strong again. When we feel broken, healing makes us whole again.

Sometimes, the best way to heal is to rest (as anyone who's broken a bone knows). To take a break from moving, thinking, and doing. To give our spirits a chance to recover from whatever is ailing us.

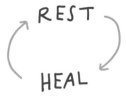

REST

HEAL

Here are a few tried-and-true ways to begin the healing process.

Journaling

Research shows that getting our thoughts and experiences on the page can help us feel better in trying times. For particularly difficult moments, there is expressive writing, a clinically based practice for processing difficult emotions and traumatic experiences. For twenty minutes a day, over the course of four days, you are prompted to examine an emotional or traumatic event through writing. Each day you go a little bit deeper in expressing your feelings. This simple practice has been proven to reduce chronic stress and anxiety and improve immunity. Although most people will feel a little sad immediately after writing, moods typically improve after an hour or so.

Although it can be particularly cathartic to write about targeted events or stressful situations, even the mere act of keeping a regular journal can be beneficial. Journaling helps us gain perspective and practice self-compassion, as we saw earlier in this chapter. Journaling offers us a safe space to explore forgiveness—of ourselves and others. Whether you choose to write every morning or turn to your journal on a whim, notice how this practice impacts your feelings, emotions, and well-being. You can start with a small journaling practice that is less structured and more free-form; the important thing is to create space for your thoughts and feelings.

Of course, healing can't be rushed: We have to be ready to process our experience in order to heal. If the mere thought of writing about a certain experience is daunting, it may be too soon to explore it in this way. If writing causes you to spiral or fixate rather than gain distance and perspective, this is also a sign to stop. Healing works best when you are ready for it.

Therapy

Sometimes it isn't enough to process challenging moments on a page. One of the most effective avenues toward healing is to engage in therapy with a seasoned practitioner and expert. Working with a licensed therapist is especially useful if you're not sure where to start on your healing journey, or if your personal challenge or trauma is interrupting or inhibiting your daily life. Therapy is a chance for you to get to know yourself, unpack your challenges, and begin to heal in ways big and small.

Cognitive behavioral therapy, or talk therapy, is my personal favorite, especially as someone who tends to process out loud. But some things are hard to put into words, and not everyone wants to talk. Luckily, there are many different forms of therapy available. Music therapy, sand therapy, art therapy, dance and movement therapy, and even animal therapy can be helpful for processing trauma and treating stress and anxiety. Each has a specific use (for example, animal therapy is particularly effective in treating social anxiety), so be sure to do your research.

If therapy is something you'd like to pursue, reach out to friends and family who may be able to recommend someone, or spend some time online researching local therapists' specialties and availability. (Be sure to check their insurance policies too.) In particular, pay attention to a therapist's areas of expertise. Although any therapist can, in theory, offer help with, say, navigating major life transitions like a career change, it's best to find someone who will be interested and prepared in your personal area of strife (for example, someone who specializes in transition anxiety, as opposed to addiction). You may also want to consider how someone's background will inform your experience in therapy; a therapist from a similar background may be able to understand more deeply what you are going through, especially if your identity is part of what brings you to therapy.

Of course, therapy can be expensive, and it takes time to find a good match (like dating, there are bound to be some awkward moments). If therapy feels out of reach or like it isn't right for you, you can still benefit from partaking in *therapeutic activities*. Many people who've never engaged in professional animal therapy will tell you that petting their dog or cat is soothing after a stressful day. Doodling, collaging, coloring books, and playing with sand can have a similarly restorative effect. Listening to music that you find comforting, energizing, or restorative can provide a calming balm, as we explored before. Dancing—or simply moving your body to a beat, sound, or rhythm, can serve as a micro-release to the day's stressors, as we learned earlier. Although working with a licensed professional is most effective, these bite-size, therapy-inspired exercises may help. They are small ways to begin to heal.

Community

For many of us, it's friends and family who lift us up when we are most down and who make our days more manageable. Having a social support network can help you cope with stress, boost your self-esteem, lower your blood pressure, enhance your mental health, and reduce feelings of emotional distress.

Although many rest practices are solo ones, you can also benefit tremendously from being an active member of a community, be it in the form of a church, sports team, drama club, knitting circle, book club, volunteer group, or any other group in which you find belonging. You might also find social support in less structured settings—grabbing lunch with a friend or coffee with a neighbor are small but effective ways of boosting your energy. (I am always amazed at what an hour of conversation with a good friend can do for my perspective, mood, and energy.) You might not "need" the company, but research shows that our experiences can be heightened in the company of others; going to the movies alone is a treat, but having someone to analyze and discuss the movie with afterward is even better. (Having company also makes comedy funnier and horror scarier.)

The next time you feel caught in a tizzy—stressed, fatigued, low, or overwhelmed—call the friend who always lifts your spirits, have a coffee break with your work wife or trusted confidant and colleague, or head to your local library or park for a dose of human interaction. With the right company, you can begin to feel better in no time.

TAKE NOTE: **Communal Mealtimes Nourish Body and Spirit**

There's a reason so many meetups, book clubs, and office meetings serve food before getting down to business. In many cultures, eating is a social act: We all need to eat, so why not share in a moment and eat together? Although it may seem more "efficient" to grab a sandwich and eat at your desk, or shovel a cereal bar in your mouth during your morning commute, there is something to be said for taking a moment to slow down and enjoy a meal and good company.

What would happen if you gave yourself the gift of pausing to eat with others? Think of all the ideas, problem-solving, relaxation, good vibes, and enthusiasm that can come out of a simple conversation over food. Mealtimes offer a lovely opportunity to nourish your body and your spirit.

Chapter 5

Ritual

Rest

MAKE REST A DAILY PRACTICE

Many of us treat rest as something we'll get to later, if we have the time. Yet for most of us, "catching up" on rest from time to time isn't enough to keep us going. Falling into a pattern of working until we are exhausted and *then* resting leaves us struggling to survive rather than thriving.

Instead, we need to build up our energy reserves over time. We need to cultivate regular rest and build habits in support of our restful pursuits. We need to learn how to quickly recover from setbacks and get back on the rest wagon as quickly as possible.

This section guides you on how to set good rest habits so that you can feel both energized and grounded throughout your days. We'll also learn best practices for recovery when, from time to time, we miss out on getting the rest we need.

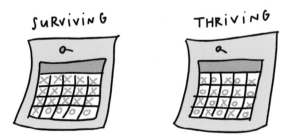

Limit

If you're reading this book, chances are that at some point in your life, you pushed past a limit and pushed yourself too far. Maybe it started for you in college, when, like so many students, you found yourself pulling all-nighters during exam season, only to crumble as soon as you got home. Perhaps you are used to working late to get a project over the finish line, despite other priorities (friends, family, or basic things like eating and sleeping) and repercussions (a nasty head cold, for one). Or maybe you've simply always felt that of everyone's needs in a group—be it a student group, a work team, a friend circle, or your own family unit—your needs come last. In each case, you learned to skirt what was comfortable and double down on work instead.

In chapters 2 and 3, we learned what blocks or causes us to ignore our own need to rest, from the cultural messages that urge us to keep going to the internal drive to do more. As we've seen, there are many forces leading us to sprint even when we ought to slow down. Luckily, no matter who we are or where we're from, limits—and the boundaries that protect them—are useful tools for ensuring we get the rest we need.

Limits tell us the points at which we cannot go further. They tell us the extent of what is possible. A limit can be physical (you can manage 10 minutes of running but not 30 minutes), emotional (you can manage one office gossip but not a culture of office toxicity), or spiritual (you believe in fate but not reincarnation). Limits can protect us from working too much, both at home and in the workplace.

Many of us have forgotten—or learned to ignore—our limits. We feel a faint headache coming on after too much screen time but swallow an Advil instead of giving our eyes a break. We insist on going to the family barbecue even if we are exhausted after a long week because we feel obliged to (or genuinely want to)—and we can relax later, right? Each time we ignore a limit, it gets harder to find the next time around.

That's why it's so important to reconnect with our limits—to remember what they are and why they're there. This isn't something you can determine by looking at how others live (which we frequently do when we compare our successes and failures against others). Our limits are highly personal—the number of hours of sleep or downtime you need every day will be different from what I need.

Examples of limits might include

- How many hours a day you are willing to work, and what those hours are

- How many social events or meetings you can manage in a day or week before becoming fatigued

- How much sleep you need

- How much alcohol you drink

- How much screen time you allow

- How much you socialize with your coworkers, neighbors, or family

	MY LIMITS	YOUR LIMITS
TARDINESS	5 MINUTES	2 HOURS
SPICY FOODS	MILD	EXTRA HOT
SOCIAL EVENTS	2 X/DAY	∞
WORK HOURS	∞	4 HRS/DAY
EXERCISE	O	∞
DOOM SCROLLING	O	∞

Reconnect with Your Limits

To reconnect with your limits, grab a notebook and pen and answer the following questions:

○ **Think back to the last time you reached a limit.** What limit did you reach? For example, perhaps a coworker scheduled a meeting with you at 5 p.m. on a Friday, but you usually stop at 4 p.m. after a long week of work.

○ **Were there any cues you reached your limit?** Cues can be physical (headaches, fatigue), emotional (irritability, a sense of dread or overwhelm), or mental (brain fog, being easily distracted).

○ **Make a list of a few other limits you remember reaching.** Keep this list as a reminder of your limits—and the physical, emotional, or mental impacts of ignoring those limits.

The Power of Boundaries

Knowing your limits means that you can begin to put boundaries in place to protect them. The right boundaries can bolster your rest rituals and efforts and protect against common rest detractors.

Establishing restful boundaries may mean setting boundaries with others—on how frequently you socialize, or tend to or take care of others. It may also require setting boundaries with yourself. As author and therapist Nedra Tawwab says, "While other people indeed have an impact on our lives, we make personal choices daily that affect the quality of our lives and who we are. With self-boundaries, we consider how *we* impact ourselves. . . . It's your responsibility to care for yourself without excuses." Setting boundaries with ourselves might include setting limits on how many hours per day we will work, making time for a variety of interests (not only our careers), turning off our devices for peace of mind, or sleeping when we are tired.

INSTEAD OF THINKING...

I WILL NOT REST UNTIL I FINISH MY TO-DO LIST

I WILL RALLY FOR THIS FAMILY EVENT NO MATTER HOW TIRED I FEEL

I WILL POWER THROUGH AT WORK

TRY...

I ACCOMPLISHED WHAT I COULD TODAY, AND THAT IS ENOUGH

I WILL BE A WARMER, MORE GENEROUS, AND HAPPIER FAMILY MEMBER IF I TAKE THE TIME I NEED TO REST INSTEAD of FORCING MYSELF TO GO

I WILL TAKE THE BREAKS I NEED TO DO GOOD WORK

With practice, setting boundaries—with ourselves and others—can get easier. In time, we may find rest is a little more in reach.

Learn to Say No

When was the last time you said "No" or "I can't" to someone as an act of self-care? Many of us are uncomfortable with saying no—we don't want to disappoint others, so we say yes to socializing, working, and taking part in activities when we'd rather be recharging with a nice bubble bath. Yet respecting our limits and setting boundaries may require us to decline invitations and activities. There may be activities, responsibilities, events, or company you need to say no to in order to say yes to rest. To prevent ourselves from giving in to non-restful activities, we need to learn to politely, firmly, and clearly say no.

Every time we say no, we reinforce our boundaries. This is as important for us as it is for others; by hearing us say no, others learn that we are committed to our boundaries, and that they are not negotiable.

Saying no can be straightforward. You can say no and explain or reiterate your boundary or simply decline without offering any reason or commitment. Sometimes, when others hear the reasons for your boundaries, they may take it as a cue to negotiate with you and try to convince you your reasons aren't valid. In this case, it may be best to simply say no without offering reasons.

Here are some examples:

○ No, I can't go out to dinner tonight; I am exhausted from a long day of childcare. (Boundary + Reason)

- No, that meeting time doesn't work for me. I only take four meetings per day. (Boundary + Commitment)

- Thank you for the invitation, but I am not up for a movie tonight. (Boundary)

SELF-REFLECT: **Check on Your Boundaries**

What boundaries—with yourself and others—might you need to set in order to get the rest you need? Thinking back to the previous exercise (page 184), make a list of possible boundaries you will uphold. According to Nedra Tawwab, boundaries that are clear and to the point work best, such as those beginning with "I want," "I need," or "I expect." For example, you might write

- I need eight hours of sleep every night.

- I want a moment to myself each morning.

- I expect my family to respect when I need some downtime.

- I expect my boss to respect my out-of-office status.

- I need to socialize with other adults once a week to maintain my sanity.

As you write these down, make note of which of these boundaries you will need to communicate to others. By communicating our needs clearly, we give others a chance to help us meet them. For self-boundaries in particular, keep this list in a handy place as a reminder of what you are committing to.

Cultivate

It's tempting to want to wait till a vacation rolls around to de-stress, relax, and feel restored. Yet research suggests that daily, continuous, habitual resting—what I call "maintenance rest"—is more impactful than intermittent "marathon rest" (such as resting on vacation or on sabbatical). When rest is part of our routine, we are able to better shield ourselves from burnout, overwhelm, and exhaustion. Frequent rest allows us to shift from playing catch-up on our energy to investing and upleveling it.

At first, this shift—both in mindset and behavior—may not come easily. As with any new endeavor, resting right takes *practice*. We can't change our relationship to rest overnight, but with dedication and the right approach, we can learn to cultivate rest every day.

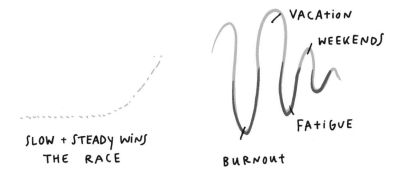

Continuous vs. Intermittent Rest

VACATION
WEEKENDS
FATIGUE

SLOW + STEADY WINS
THE RACE

BURNOUT

How to Make Rest a Regular Habit

The more rest is ingrained in our daily lives, the more likely we are to stick with it and the more readily we'll be able to reap its benefits. The following pages will help you develop good rest habits and cultivate regular rest. When it comes to starting a new habit, there are a few rules of thumb to keep in mind.

Start on the Right Foot

According to research from behavioral economist Dr. Katy Milkman, your odds of forming good habits improve if you take advantage of "the fresh-start effect." Certain days—like the first day of the week, month, or year; the beginning of a season; and birthdays—act as a mental reset button and give you an edge for starting a new habit. On these days, you can set aside the "old" you and make way for a new, better version of yourself because you have the impression that anything is possible. (If you've ever set a New Year's resolution or done spring-cleaning on the first day of the season, you know what I mean.) A fresh start is more motivating, and less daunting, than starting on any old Wednesday.

Milkman's research suggests that life milestones like becoming a parent, getting a promotion, becoming ill, or moving cross-country—or even smaller events like trying a new coffee shop or gym—can similarly serve to clean the slate. These moments offer what Milkman calls "psychological do-overs" that create a fundamental shift in your identity. (The same moments, however, can upend existing routines and rituals, so it's best not to indiscriminately pursue major life changes unless you are ready to adapt in both directions.)

As you think about the resting habits you wish to form, consider whether the moment is right. Search for a fresh start to give your efforts a boost. How might you get started on the right foot?

Start Small

Starting a new habit often comes with a welcome surge of energy and motivation. But in our excitement, we can sometimes swing too big and miss. In the beginning, even a small miss can damage our confidence and derail our progress.

To give yourself the best shot at success, break large, ambitious goals and projects into smaller, more manageable ones. This ensures we don't bite off more than we can chew and gives us a road map for making incremental progress toward the finish line.

One simple way of starting small is to follow what habit expert James Clear calls "the two-minute rule." This means breaking down the habit you want to start into its smallest version, or something that can be done in under two minutes. For example, if the resting habit you'd like to cultivate is to read a book before going to bed (as part of your new winding-down routine), you might start by reading one page each night instead of an entire chapter. Or, if you'd like to get into the practice of taking naps in the afternoon, start by simply closing your eyes for two minutes. By breaking things down into smaller chunks, they become more achievable.

Make it Specific

Research shows that the more specific your habit, the better your chances are of setting and maintaining it. That means it isn't enough to say "I want to rest more." (Don't worry, that was my first draft too.) Instead, you have to get specific. James Clear suggests including the behavior, a time, and a location. Saying "I'm going to be in bed before 10 p.m., five days a week, on weekdays" is specific and actionable.

Watch Your Language

How we talk about our new rest habits matters. According to author and habit expert Gretchen Rubin, habits are more likely to stick when we use words that empower rather than disempower us. For example, the following phrases use empowering language:

o   I don't . . . (stay up late at night)

o   I choose to . . . (go to bed early)

- ○ I'm going to . . . (put down my phone)

- ○ I don't want to . . . (wake up with a hangover)

The same habits are less likely to stick when we use disempowering language, such as:

- ○ I can't . . . (watch Netflix anymore)

- ○ I'm not allowed to . . . (have wine at dinner)

- ○ I'm supposed to . . . (meditate)

Play the Part

It's easy to get in your own way on your journey to rest, particularly if you come with negative beliefs and expectations about what you are capable of. If you are stuck in an identity that isn't serving you, such as "workaholic" or "perfectionist," you'll need to play a different part ("rest guru," anyone?). To do this, you need to shift your beliefs as well as your behaviors. James Clear suggests the following:

- ○ Decide the type of person you want to be.

- ○ Prove it to yourself with small wins.

By "wins," Clear means taking actions or steps that are in line with the person you want to become. Each action is a "vote" for the person you want to be—and evidence that you are becoming that person.

To become a person who prioritizes rest, you need to play the part through your actions. Every time you follow through and take a calming walk outside, go to bed on time, journal, play, or embrace solitude and quiet, you "cast a vote" that you are a person who prioritizes rest.

Poet Maggie Smith shares a similar sentiment in her book of affirmations, *Keep Moving*. "Close the gap between yourself and your spirit, the person you know you can be," she writes. "Let your choices reflect the person you want to become, not just the person you think you are."

SELF-REFLECT: **Let Go of Old Stories**

We all have personal narratives and beliefs we hold within us. Sometimes these are empowering, but other times they are limiting. To give yourself the best chance at rest, it's time to shed any limiting stories and write some new ones.

- What stories have you internalized about yourself that may be getting in the way of cultivating good rest habits? For example, you might consider yourself a perfectionist, pride yourself on being a workaholic, or even fancy yourself the life of the party.

- What do you want your rest narrative to be? Notice whether this is different from how you currently see yourself. Might any of those old messages need reframing?

- How might you "cast your vote" through actions and behaviors that support this new narrative?

Make It Rewarding

Like so many of us, I've known for years that good sleep hygiene includes keeping screens out of the bedroom, but that hadn't stopped me from checking email or watching one last episode in bed until recently. Why couldn't I do what I knew was good for me? Because, quite simply, it was more pleasurable to watch TV than to power down. Even though I knew I'd suffer the consequences the next day, the short-term payoff was too great to ignore.

This is the problem of present bias, or the tendency to favor instant gratification over long-term rewards. This bias is the reason so many of us drink more alcohol than we should (getting buzzed is a short-term reward that beats the long-term reward of not having a hangover), smoke (we favor short-term stress relief over the long-term reward of a lower risk of lung cancer), and put off rest even when we want it (we indulge in "me time" scrolling social media at the end of a long day rather than being mindful of the long-term reward of feeling better rested tomorrow). One of the biggest challenges to forming habits that stick is that there are a million other things that we could be doing that would frankly be a lot more fun.

Dr. Katy Milkman describes our options in terms of "wants" versus "shoulds." "Wants" may give us immediate pleasure but have little long-term value, whereas "shoulds" offer less benefit in the near term and more in the long run. "Going to bed early versus going to bed late and watching TV is a want, because in the moment that'll be fun, but in the long run you'll regret it," she says.

To make a habit stick, you have to add some short-term pleasure to the mix. As Mary Poppins says, "A spoonful of sugar helps the medicine go down." Here are some ways to mix in some fun as you form a rest habit.

Pair It

When it's hard to start a new habit, it can help to pair it with an existing habit—especially one you already enjoy. For example, instead of saying "I resolve to exercise more," you might try pairing it with something pleasurable, like listening to podcasts (assuming that's fun for you). A good pairing might sound like: "I'll only binge true-crime podcasts while I exercise." Pairing can also be used to cut back on harmful habits. If you want to watch less TV, a paired habit could be: "I will only watch TV while folding laundry." This is called temptation bundling—linking something you want to do with something you need to do.

You can also pair activities by using cue-based planning. For example, if you find yourself putting off sleep at bedtime, you might tell yourself, "When I finish clearing the dinner table, I will get into my pajamas." Clearing the table is now your cue for starting your bedtime routine. Or, if you're struggling to develop a new daily journaling practice, you can pair it with an existing daily habit, like eating breakfast. "Journal every day" thus becomes "journal for five minutes every day after breakfast." Breakfast becomes an anchor for your new practice. In each case, you're taking an everyday, ordinary activity and using it to tee up a new, restful one.

Invite a Friend

Not every resting activity benefits from company (in fact, many of us find solitude to be the most restful of all), but some things are simply more fun in the company of others. For example, many people struggle to do a tech shabbat (see pages 55–59) on their own, but partnering with friends and family can make the event festive and easier to commit to. If your motivation is lagging, look for a resting practice where you can invite a friend, partner, or colleague to join you. Not only will it be more fun, but it also keeps you accountable to following through, since you won't be going it alone. More on that next.

Use Cue-Based Planning to Start a New Rest Routine

What is a specific resting habit you would like to cultivate? What is a reliable routine or ritual you can pair it with? For example, if you're looking to cut down on phone use for peace of mind, could you turn your phone off when you get home and take off your shoes? What will serve as your cue? Write this down on a sticky note and leave it in a visible place, like a bathroom mirror. Try putting your cue-based planning into action this week.

Create Accountability

If a habit falls in the forest, and no one is around to hear it, does it make a sound? Some of us find setting new habits easy (these folks usually score high on conscientiousness on personality tests, and love New Year's resolutions). But most of us do not fall into this category. Sometimes we need a little help—a little accountability—in our efforts to rest more.

Accountability can come in many forms: deadlines (boring but helpful for keeping us on track), friends (it's harder to flake out on yoga class if you've committed to going with a friend), community (knowing you are not alone motivates you to keep going), going public with your intentions (sharing with your personal network or writing about your efforts online), or even tracking your progress (counting and keeping streaks for good behavior). Depending on your personality, some forms of accountability may make you cringe (personally, the idea of keeping a streak sounds terrible to me). Pick what feels fun and easy to *you*.

Make It Convenient

Many of us believe that if we can summon enough self-discipline, we can resist answering that email or scrolling social media again. When we cannot, we take these failings personally: Our failure to abstain and make change must mean something is wrong with us.

Yet research from social psychologist Dr. Wendy Wood shows that strong intentions and willpower can only take us so far. "Decision and will simply aren't the tools to use for making continued sacrifices in order to persist at our new goals," she writes. Believing that good intentions paired with self-discipline (also known as the "strong intentions and willpower theory of self-change") will help us break our phone-checking habit and build a meditation practice is a recipe for disappointment.

Instead, you can encourage rest by making restful habits convenient and bad habits inconvenient. To make non-restful habits inconvenient, you might raise the "cost" of them. For example, charging our phone outside our bedroom raises the "cost" of aimlessly scrolling on it at night; by making it more inconvenient for us to use our phones in bed, we make it easier to keep good sleep hygiene and get the rest we need. Here are two shortcuts to making rest more convenient.

Use Visual Cues

Visual cues support your restful habits by reminding you of your mission to rest and making it easy to execute. Take these, for example:

o   If you want to succeed at your tech shabbat, you can gather all devices and keep them out of sight for the day.

o   If you want to stick to your bedtime routine, you can put a good book and your favorite pajamas on your bed an hour before bedtime.

o   If you want to turn rest into a ritual, you can create a cozy corner specifically for that purpose, or use a favorite chair for reading or relaxing.

Make the Decision Once

Many of us engage in trade-off thinking, mentally weighing trade-offs that take us out of rest mode. For example, while resting, we may feel as though we should be working; while working, we may resent missing out on rest time. In each case, we are thinking about what we "could" be doing if we weren't already occupied.

This kind of thinking is not only distracting but mentally taxing. Double- or even triple-processing our decisions hurts our executive functioning, including our ability to reason, think rationally, exercise willpower, and make good decisions. When we are cognitively fatigued, making good, restful decisions can be difficult.

Instead, we need to reduce second-guessing our commitments to rest as much as possible. One way to do this is to streamline decision-making. We want to reduce what economist Dr. Eldar Shafir and psychologist Dr. Sendhil Mullainathan call vigilance choices (which require ongoing monitoring and repeated decision-making) and rely instead on one-off choices (which require a single decision and are thus easier to maintain). The less decision-making, the better. (A true habit is, after all, ultimately made without thinking.) The tech shabbat is effective for this reason; once the decision has been made to take the day off from technology, the rest of the day's decisions fall in line. Because it is a recurring event, no additional planning or decision-making is needed.

In practice, that might mean signing up for a *regular* restful activity— say, a weekly drawing class (one decision)—rather than having to plan, negotiate, and carve out time each week for a new leisure activity (many decisions). Or it might mean cutting your Netflix subscription (one decision) rather than having to decide every night to not fall down a TV rabbit hole (many decisions).

Make It a Regular Event
A behavior is considered a habit when it becomes automatic. This happens largely through repetition: The more you repeat the behavior, the

more it becomes second nature. Each time we repeat it, we strengthen the brain's association with it, making it easier, more effective, and more efficient to complete over time. In other words, the longer you've done something, the more of a habit it becomes. This process can take two to three months, but it's worth putting in the work up front to make it easier to rest down the line.

Give Yourself a Pass (But Just One)

Falling off the wagon is a predictable part of the habit-making and habit-keeping process. (Holidays and vacations in particular are common culprits.) It is best to know this up front, so that when a setback does occur, you don't spend time berating yourself.

To quickly recover from unavoidable setbacks, practice self-compassion when they occur. Understand that this is all part of the process of growth and change. Once you've given yourself the permission to be human and make mistakes, get back into the ring and try again. Do your best not to let these misses accumulate—research shows that the further back you fall, the harder it is to recover and regain momentum in making change. "If you fall off the wagon, get right back on it," says Dr. Katy Milkman.

Remember the Basics

Setbacks can make us feel as if we are starting over. This can feel daunting and discouraging: All that progress, out the window! In these moments, remember how you first began your restful habits. Perhaps you looked for fresh starts to get off on the right foot. You may have tried the two-minute rule as a small start to a bigger resting routine. These tools are especially helpful for getting back on track. And remember: Not all progress is visible. Setbacks are a necessary part of the journey.

Outline Your Rest Plan

To create a personalized rest plan, consider the following:

○ **Which rest habit will you start with?** Be specific. For example, "go to bed by 10 p.m. three days a week" is clearer and more actionable than "go to bed earlier."

○ **Who or what will help you commit?** For example, will you have an accountability partner or friend group by your side?

○ **What strategies will you rely on?** Perhaps you can sweeten the deal Mary Poppins–style or find a routine to pair your new habit with.

○ **When can you start?** Remember to consider fresh starts, from the first day of spring to your first day at a new job.

Recover

Although making a regular habit of rest is our best chance at feeling well-rested, energized, and inspired, sometimes we push ourselves too far and neglect to give ourselves the care we deserve. Luckily, there are three recovery methods to get back to our pre-stress baseline: maintenance rest (evening and weekend rest), marathon rest (vacations and sabbaticals) and in-the-moment rest (quick microbreaks to get us back on track).

Maintenance Rest

Research from organizational psychologists like Dr. Sabine Sonnentag suggests that with a few simple practices, you can make your leisure time more restful. These techniques are particularly useful for everyday evening recovery, and they can aid in sleep and feeling well-rested the next day.

The following guidelines will help you pick the right evening activity. You can use the same advice to maximize your weekend rest, too.

○ **Try "low-duty" activities, not "high-duty" ones, to aid in your recovery.** High-duty activities include life admin, childcare, and household tasks. Low-duty activities include socializing, hobbies, creative pursuits, and exercise. We all have chores to catch up on, but as we learned in chapter 4, it's also important to play. Not only is engaging in low-duty activities more fun, but intentionally prioritizing these reinforces our personal sense of agency, which in turn helps us to feel more grounded. Feeling in control of how we spend our leisure time makes these activities more calming and restorative.

○ **Choose activities that facilitate psychological detachment, or not thinking about work.** If we are grocery shopping and mentally composing an email to our boss at the same time, it will be difficult to recover from our work stress (we're still in it!). Find activities that help you gain distance from your work (for me, reading fiction seems to help), and once you've left work, put (and keep!) your work devices away.

○ **Think relaxing, not activating.** Look for activities that encourage relaxation—yoga, gentle movement, puzzles, knitting, massage, or napping—rather than activities that further stimulate your fight-or-flight stress response. We want to get back to our pre-stress baseline, not exacerbate it.

Marathon Rest (Vacations and Sabbaticals)

When burnout and fatigue hit, "marathon" resting sessions like vacations, and, if we are lucky, sabbaticals, can help. Just be careful not to fall into a cycle of burnout → marathon rest → burnout. Vacations and sabbaticals can help us recover but will always be more restorative if we're starting from a place of wellness, not burnout. (Vacation benefits also tend to fade quickly, as anyone on their first day back at work after a break can attest to.)

In addition to taking care to pick the right restful activities (the guidelines for evening rest work well here too), you can also try the following.

Ease into Your Vacations

Give yourself a buffer day (or more) to get into the vacation spirit. It can be difficult to abruptly change from work (stress) mode to vacation (relaxation) mode. Take it slow on the first few days of your vacation, knowing it may take you a moment to mentally unplug. You might also consider leaving for your vacations midweek and returning midweek: A midweek journey is likely to be less crowded and chaotic (fewer people at the airport, fewer cars on the road, etc.), and more relaxing. Returning to a half week of work instead of a full one also offers a more gentle transition back to reality after vacation.

Be wary of overplanning. Some people love to plan every minute of their weekend or vacation, but remember: The point is to have fun and relax. For many of us, a packed itinerary sounds good ahead of time, but stressful the day of. (If you are the exception, go forth and enjoy that busy schedule.)

Microbreaks

Sometimes we don't have time for a marathon resting session, and an evening recovery session is too far off. If our stress or fatigue begins to get the best of us, recovery can't wait. Whether you're feeling sluggish from the afternoon slump or anxious thanks to a surprise one-on-one with your boss, a microbreak can help get you back on track. Research from organizational psychologists shows that the most impactful breaks for replenishing our cup are frequent, take place outdoors, and include movement, intention, and socializing.

Unfortunately, many of our usual go-to "breaks" (scrolling on social media, catching up on work emails, watching TV) fail to check all the boxes (or any of them). These are typically solo activities that involve little to no movement, frequently take place inside, and fail to make us feel more rested. A quick walk outside with a friend is much closer to the ideal break.

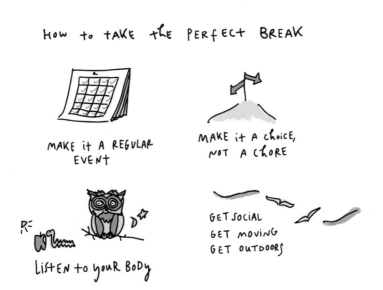

HOW to tAKE the PERfECt BREAK

MAKE it A REGULAR EVENt

MAKE it A choicE, NOT A CHoRE

LiStEN to youR BoDy

GET SOCiAL
GET MoViNG
GET OUTDooRS

Identify Your Natural Rest Cycle

If you've ever found yourself rereading the same sentence for ten minutes or taking too long to send a simple email, it may be that you're trying (unsuccessfully) to push through your natural rest time. What would happen if you were able to recognize your rest cycle and honor it instead?

Follow these steps to find your natural rest cycle:

○ **Are you a night owl or an early bird?** These are chronotypes—typologies that describe our natural rhythm of energy and sleep needs throughout a given day. Early birds are most alert in the morning, while night owls come alive after dark. Each of us has a specific chronotype, influenced by both our environment and our age. (A lot of us are night owls as teens and early birds at sixty.) Which are you?

○ **On a typical day, when does your energy flag?** A typical rhythm looks like this: alertness and productivity (for 90 to 120 minutes) followed by fatigue, rest, and recovery (for approximately 20 minutes). This is known as the basic rest–activity cycle, an ultradian rhythm that manages energy production, output, and recovery multiple times a day. On an average wake schedule, we usually feel dips around midmorning and midafternoon. Make note of when your energy peaks and valleys typically occur.

○ **Plan the day—and its breaks— accordingly.** Given what you have learned, you can design your day in line with your natural rest cycle, rather than fight against it. If you know when your energy usually dips, rather than gulping down another cup of coffee and powering through,

you can honor this cycle by resting instead. That might mean adjusting your wake and sleep schedules, taking a power nap, going for a walk, or even taking a few deep breaths or a minute of silence and solitude. If you're tempted to power through, keep in mind that the more we ignore our need for rest and recovery, the worse our productivity and energy become. Instead of charging ahead, it's best to follow your rhythm and take a break. Now that you know your natural rest cycle, what would an ideal day look like for you?

Invite

Abundance

I 'm sitting in a coffee shop, a cup of tea in my hands and a stack of library books at my side. Tonight, I will pick a book from my pile and find myself transported to a faraway place. I will fall asleep easily, and though I'll likely be woken up by my son, who is still learning to sleep independently, I will have gone to bed happy. For now, I watch the sunlight stream through the window and the neighborhood come to life. From my perch I see friends meeting up on the corner, dogs marking a beloved hydrant, and children squealing on scooters with parents hurrying behind them.

Only half an hour earlier, I was on the verge of losing it. After multiple loads of laundry, packing, and organizing before our upcoming move, I could tell I needed a break. I needed to stop sorting and organizing, to stop corralling my son into his clothes or whisking our barking dog away from the front door every time a neighbor walked by.

Before, I would have powered through—kept packing and watching the kiddo, walked the dog, managed one responsibility after another. But the work I have done this year—this year of experimenting with rest and relaxation, of building my understanding of how to rest in a way that is restful *to me*—is starting to pay off. I am getting better at recognizing what stress feels like in my body, at sensing frustration and overwhelm on the horizon. I have a better idea of what I need, and I'm practicing getting it every day.

Frazzled but not yet entirely overwhelmed, I said to my husband, "I need a moment to myself." "Great," he told me. He, too, is happy I haven't lost it yet. He clicked into "go" mode and quickly (or as quickly as one can with a toddler in tow) vacated the apartment with my son. They were off to their adventure and I to mine.

I didn't go to a reiki session or book a last-minute massage. I didn't try a new rest experiment, like a salt cave, energy medicine, acupuncture, or any others on my list. I tried something much simpler: I closed my eyes for a few minutes and listened to the sound of my breath. Eventually, gradually, I gathered my things to visit the library. I wandered the stacks, scanning the spines and letting the titles speak to me. I judged each book by its cover, like I always do, and emerged armed with a stack of books I can't wait to read. I ambled over to a local coffee shop and got comfy.

It's nothing special. But for me, that's what makes it so special. My husband has given me the morning to rest while he watches our toddler, and I am happy.

Final Rest Revelations

What would you do with a morning to yourself to relax? The rest practices that work best for you will undoubtedly be different from mine—unique, as they should be, to your personal experience. As you embark on your own rest journey, here are seven final rest revelations to help you on your way.

Rest Is Simple

When I first began my year of rest research and exploration, it was
the pampering I most looked forward to—the special visits to a spa or
studio that would send me into a state of curated bliss. But what really
made a difference were far more mundane experiments, like setting a
bedtime and sticking to it, cutting out caffeine, and skipping the glass
of wine at dinner, save for special occasions. I learned to enjoy the daily
drive to pick my son up from school, using it as a dedicated space for
mind-wandering. I reconnected with my lost love of reading—not for
research, but solely for the pleasure of it. I remembered to take a
moment to look at the leaves rustling in the trees and listen to the birds
singing outside my window. I began to look for fractal patterns wherever I went. These were simple, restful practices I could do every day.
As you embark upon your own rest journey, remember that sometimes
the most restful activities are the simplest. If you can fit these activities in your day-to-day, you can make meaningful, restorative change
over time.

Rest Is Intuitive

In my research, many rest-seekers confessed that they simply didn't
know *how* to rest. I felt this way too. What *was* rest? How did it work?
I could not rest until I found the answer. (Hence, this book.) But truthfully, rest would have come sooner and more easily if I'd simply trusted
myself in the process.

We were made for rest. It's why we nod off when we are tired and why
our mind wanders without our permission. It is why we feel at peace
at the sight of a magical vista or sunset, and why it's much easier to
be present when our hearts are full. Though it can feel as if we don't
know how to rest, if there's one thing I've learned over the course of

researching this book, it's that we have most of what we need within us already.

Like using a muscle that's atrophied, resting can feel awkward in the beginning. But trust that your mind and body know what to do. The more you rest, the more your mind and body remember, and the quicker you can reap the benefits of deep, luscious rest. Trust your intuitions about rest.

Rest Is Going at Your Own Pace

Throughout my year of rest research, my characteristic intensity and eagerness surfaced again and again. I raced to find rest techniques that might work for me and jammed my calendar full of rest experiments. (This turned out to be more stressful than restful.) I devoted myself to the cause, sometimes taking advice to the extreme, like when I stopped (instead of simply reducing with intention) taking phone calls, listening to podcasts, or listening to the radio in an attempt to quiet my mind, as if that might help me recover sooner. (It didn't.) The more I rushed and the harder I tried to uncover the secret to rest, the more I felt behind, wondering when I would finally, mercifully, crack the tough nut that rest was turning out to be.

Eventually, I slowed down. I let go of my inner urgency, high expectations, and rigid rules. That's when I started making progress.

Rest does not come through sheer force or will, but must be courted, gently, slowly, patiently. That means trying new things with ease, not hurry. It means taking small steps before giant ones. It means pacing ourselves to find what works for us.

As you embrace a life of rest, remember that you are on a journey. Try not to stress about progress, setbacks, or struggles, or compare yourself to others. Ease into your experimentation. Lower your expectations for how quickly you will recover from your exhaustion. Accept what is possible day by day. Take it slow and allow rest to come to you. Give yourself the time and space to build a more rested life. Like the tortoise and the hare teach us, slow and steady wins the race.

Remember, too, that rest is not all or nothing. What we need will be different from one day to the next. All we can do is try to find balance and grace in our actions, and breathe through the rest.

Rest Is Guilt-Free

For me, prioritizing rest has meant not just finding the right activities, but also the right feelings. It's meant taking time to myself without feeling guilty—no small feat. I've learned that taking a break to read a book, take a walk, watch the clouds, or listen to a podcast doesn't make me a bad parent, friend, spouse, or daughter. More and more, I understand that it's better for everyone—myself, my family, my friends, even my work—if I put on my own oxygen mask first. Taking care of myself is a gift for all of us. Recognizing this—and believing it—is a small but important step toward treating myself not as a robot or machine, but as a human being with her own wants and needs.

As you experiment with how to incorporate rest into your own routine, remember not to let feelings of guilt derail your progress. It may help to share your feelings with others, like the spouse, child, or friend you are scared to let down. You might find that your fears are unwarranted, and that there's nothing to feel guilty about after all. Your support circle might even be ready and eager to help you on your quest for rest.

Rest Is Community

Some rest techniques are more bang for their buck than others. I had always thought of getting help with childcare as a means to other things, like working, cooking, *doing*. Yet it has completely changed my relationship to rest. Getting childcare (an obvious act of self-care in retrospect) made rest possible.

Sometimes, to get the rest we need, we need help—in the form of babysitters and daycare, paid time off, and neighbors and friends who drop off soup and takeout when we're recovering from a bad cold or surgery. Your ability to rest is not entirely contingent on *you*. We all need help—from our families, communities, neighbors, employers, and government—to get the rest we need.

Learn to ask for the help you need from others. It will dictate the kinds of jobs you take, the friends you make, and the rest you get. You may be surprised by how much others want to help you.

Rest Is Staying Curious (and Persistent)

Throughout my year of experimentation, I hit many dead ends. There were practices I failed to appreciate or understand (like ASMR), and others that simply didn't deliver on their promise of relaxation (like salt cave therapy). But no matter the result, I never regretted trying these out.

Whether a given tactic fit or failed was in some ways beside the point, because either way, the experience taught me something new about what I needed to feel rested. I learned that I prefer rest practices involving physical touch (like reiki or massage) more than those promising mental relaxation. (For me, the physical release usually led to a quieting of the mind.) I learned that small versions of big practices were equally powerful, and that, even if I couldn't master the power nap, I could feel rested just from closing my eyes for a few minutes. I had to stay open-minded and curious (and persistent) to figure this out. I had to be willing to experiment—and fail—to find what worked for me. After all, experimentation leads to discovery.

I hope you take that same spirit of openness and experimentation to your own pursuit of rest. If we are too quick to judge or quit too soon, we'll never find the best rest activities for us. As you explore which rest techniques work for you, remember to stay curious and keep exploring.

Rest Is Change

As we saw in chapter 2, our ability to rest hinges on far more than the individual. This is why it's so important to agitate for change—not just in ourselves, but also in our offices, schools, and communities.

You might not consider yourself to be a contrarian, protester, dissenter, or activist, but aspiring to a lifestyle of rest *does* go against the popular majority and the message that work—not rest—is best. You can be a change agent by prioritizing rest in your own life. Be intentional about how you model rest and work for your children, coworkers, and communities. You can also advocate for change by donating to organizations that champion restful causes, voting for candidates who support policies that make rest possible, and speaking up about the importance of rest. Do your best to keep going, even if it sometimes means swimming upstream.

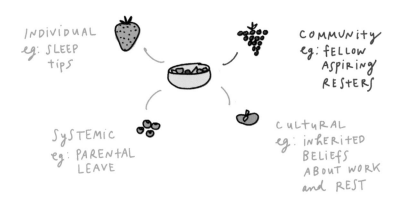

INGREDIENTS for RESTFUL CHANGE

INDIVIDUAL
eg: SLEEP
tips

COMMUNITY
eg: FELLOW
ASPIRING
RESTERS

SYSTEMIC
eg: PARENTAL
LEAVE

CULTURAL
eg: INHERITED
BELIEFS
ABOUT WORK
and REST

Make Rest Visible

When we prioritize rest, we can't see our progress in the same way we can see hours logged at work, promotions and accolades earned, to-dos checked off a list, or a perfectly cleaned house after a day of decluttering. At first glance, it's hard to see rest's impact.

Yet when we don't rest, we feel the effects immediately. When we wake up tired day after day, or can't seem to focus no matter how hard we try, or feel a low-grade tension looming over us wherever we go, we know we haven't rested enough. When we snap at our partners or are short-tempered with our coworkers, we know our rest reserves are low. Some of us catch on quicker than others, but eventually—after an adult tantrum, meltdown, or stress fest—it's obvious we're not well rested.

Rest *is* making an impact—on our work, in our creativity, in how we show up for ourselves and others. We know this when we wake up energized and content. We know it when we meet others with generosity and patience (even when they are grumpy). We know it when we are able to show ourselves self-compassion for mistakes made, or regulate our emotions after a stressful encounter. We know it when we feel good—creative, open, happy—in our hearts, minds, and bodies. Even if we can't see it, we can *feel* the effects of rest. Rest is the invisible force that helps us feel calmness, love, joy, peace, and energy in our lives.

We need to make rest more visible in our own lives. Notice when you are doing something restful—a luxurious nap, a brief moment to watch the sunset, a relaxing night with friends and family—and celebrate it. Recognize how *good* rest makes you feel. Notice the abundance rest brings into your life. Enjoy yourself freely as you rest, knowing its benefits spill over from you to those you love. Be still or move your body however feels good to you. Pay attention to all the good that rest brings to you. Savor the feeling. Do it again.

As you notice the positive changes in your own life, tell a friend. Share this book. Inspire others to take back the reins of rest and discover what gives them joy, calm, and peace. Show others what is possible.

In times when you are not sure your rest efforts are working, remind yourself: "I cannot see it *yet*, but I will feel it soon."

Acknowledgments

Throughout my rest journey, there were many people who in small and big ways helped to bring calm, ease, and joy to my life—and who helped me write this book.

I am grateful to the many experts who personally shared their insight and advice on getting rest with me and provided crucial introductions for more research: Katy Milkman, Daniel Jin Blum, Kin Yuen, Anna Codrea-Rado, Lavender Suarez, Rob Walker, Meredith Arthur, Zee Clarke, Darby Saxbe, and Eve Rodsky.

To my community of fellow aspiring resters and user research participants, thank you for sharing your stories with me. Thank you also to everyone who tested my rest exercises and helped me refine them. A special shout-out to my uncle, Russell Gordon, the most loyal of them all, who tested every single one.

To my early readers—Nicole Gulotta for helping me see the forest for the trees, Jenny Blake for reminding me to bring in some sunshine, Melody Wilding for helping keep exercises fresh and actionable, and Dolly Chugh for bringing a sensitive eye to a pivotal chapter—thank you for making this book better.

Special thanks, as always, to my agent, Leila Campoli, who believed in this story from the jump and helped me find a home at Chronicle Books. To my team at Chronicle: Rachel Hiles, Katie van Amburg, Sarah Billingsley, Lizzie Vaughan, and Wynne Au-Yeung, thank you for helping this book come to life, and beautifully! Working with such a talented team made things so calm and restful.

Thanks to anyone who gave a "hell yes" or a "I need this book now" vote of confidence in the book's early stages. Thank you also to my author's group, for providing inspiration and good company along the way. To Alex Elle, for the beautiful foreword and for the writing check-ins.

Finally, to my family, for reminding me to slow down and for giving me the space to recover when I need it. To the Abuelos, primos, tíos and tías, Raquel, Russell, Ann, and Dane, thank you for offering a quiet space to write—and babysitting, too. Special thanks to Isaac and Elio—I think we did it better this time around.

Notes

Introduction

Page 12: In Hong Kong, you can pay to take a "sleeping bus tour": Alice Fung and Matthew Cheng, "People Are Paying to Sleep on a Bus for 5 Hours. It's Called a 'Sleeping Bus Tour'," *USA Today*, October 22, 2021, https://www.usatoday.com/story/news/world/2021/10/22/hong-kong-company-launches-sleep-bus-tour/6133398001/.

Page 12: In China, the tang ping, or "lying flat," movement has taken hold among young workers: Ivana Davidovic, "'Lying flat': Why some Chinese are putting work second," *BBC News*, February 16, 2022, https://www.bbc.com/news/business-60353916.

Page 13: Other Chinese workers partake in an activity that has resonated worldwide, "revenge bedtime procrastination": Lu-Hai Liang, "The Psychology Behind 'Revenge Bedtime Procrastination,'" *BBC News*, November 25, 2020, https://www.bbc.com/worklife/article/20201123-the-psychology-behind-revenge-bedtime-procrastination.

For more on this phenomenon, see: Eric Suni, "What Is 'Revenge Bedtime Procrastination'?", *Sleep Foundation*, August 29, 2022, https://www.sleepfoundation.org/sleep-hygiene/revenge-bedtime-procrastination.

Page 13: Research from the World Health Organization shows that death by overwork has spread beyond Japan's borders: "Long working hours increasing deaths from heart disease and stroke: WHO, ILO," *World Health Organization*, May 27, 2021, https://www.who.int/news/item/17-05-2021-long-working-hours-increasing-deaths-from-heart-disease-and-stroke-who-ilo.

Page 21: Other circumstances, such as your mental health, will also inform which practices are most useful to you: Our mental health and physical health both play a major role in how rested we feel. Consider this book a starting point for deeper exploration and discussion. The goal is to help you feel more energized and centered.

Chapter 1

Page 35: Burnout has three parts: "Burn-out an 'occupational phenomenon': International Classification of Diseases," *World Health Organization*, May 28, 2019, https://www.who.int/news/item/28-05-2019-burn-out-an-occupational-phenomenon-international-classification-of-diseases.

Page 36: According to a 2022 Ohio State University study, 66 percent of working parents are burned out: "New report finds burnout among working parents associated with more mental health concerns, punitive behavior toward children," May 5, 2022, https://nursing.osu.edu/news/2022/05/05/new-report-finds-burnout-among-working-parents-associated-more-mental-health.

Chapter 2

Page 49: It's more productive—and restful—to simply focus on one thing at a time: Daniel Levitin, *The Organized Mind*, (New York: Dutton, 2014), 16.

Page 50: Data from one of the earliest trials, in Iceland, is particularly encouraging: Guðmundur D. Haraldsson and Jack Kellam, "Going Public: Iceland's Journey to a Shorter Working week," *Autonomy*, July 4, 2021, https://autonomy.work/portfolio/icelandsww.

Page 52: Social media tends to edit out the realities: For more, see Kathryn Jezer-Morton, "Nuke It from Orbit," *Mothers Under the Influence*, February 2, 2022, https://mothersundertheinfluence.substack.com/p/nuke-it-from-orbit.

Page 52: Statistically speaking, the birth of a first child is even a risk factor for divorce: Molly Millwood, *To Have and to Hold: Motherhood, Marriage, and the Modern Dilemma* (New York: Harper Wave, 2019), 137–138.

Page 60: This is especially true for those of us whose identities are at the intersection of multiple marginalized communities: For more information, see the theory of intersectionality by Kimberlé Crenshaw.

Page 62: "My heart rate shoots up": Zee Clarke, "Grocery Shopping While Black," *Medium*, July 12, 2018, https://medium.com /@zhalisaclarke/grocery-shopping-while-black -655689c9fb2e.

Page 63: People who experience discrimination, racism, and prejudice face many negative health consequences: Jenna Wortham, "Racism's Psychological Toll," *New York Times*, June 24, 2015, https://www.nytimes.com/2015/06/24 /magazine/racisms-psychological-toll.html.

Page 63: Discrimination and microaggressions can set off the body's alarm system, raising blood pressure and cortisol levels: Isabel Wilkerson, *Caste: The Origins of Our Discontents* (New York: Random House, 2020), 304.

Page 63: People of color at the top of their field: Wilkerson, *Caste: The Origins of Our Discontents*, 306–307.

Page 64: "If you want to understand the poor, imagine yourself with your mind elsewhere": Shafir Eldar and Sendhil Mullainathan, *Scarcity: The New Science of Having Less and How It Defines Our Lives* (New York: Picador/Henry Holt and Company, 2014), 161.

Page 64: Impoverished people have "lower effective capacity" than the rich: Eldar and Mullainathan, *Scarcity: The New Science of Having Less and How It Defines Our Lives*, 161.

Page 66: Though many women are desperate for "me time," it's usually the first thing cut from their busy schedules: Brigid Schulte, *Overwhelmed: Work, Love, and Play When No One Has the Time* (New York: Sarah Crichton Books, Farrar, Straus and Giroux, 2014), 29.

Chapter 3

Page 79: You are not doomed to a life without rest if you're naturally high-strung or prone to workaholism: Workaholism is more than enthusiasm or passion for your work; it is considered to be closer to that of an addiction. It is more common in private sectors and the self-employed, along with highly educated workers and managers. Workaholism is not a clinical diagnosis, but studies have shown that it is positively linked with psychiatric symptoms of ADHD, OCD, and anxiety. For more

information, see: Cecilie Schou Andreassen, Mark D. Griffiths, Rajita Sinha, Jørn Hetland, and Ståle Pallesen, "The Relationships Between Workaholism and Symptoms of Psychiatric Disorders: A Large-Scale Cross-Sectional Study," *PLoS One* 11, no. 5 (May 2016): e0152978, doi: 10.1371/journal.pone .0152978.

Page 87: "The question I'm asked most often": Nedra Glover Tawwab, *Set Boundaries, Find Peace: A Guide to Reclaiming Yourself* (New York: TarcherPerigee, 2021), 106.

Page 91: Our sense of smell is uniquely linked to the hippocampus: Wendy Suzuki and Billie Fitzpatrick, *Good Anxiety: Harnessing the Power of the Most Misunderstood Emotion* (New York: Atria Books, 2021), 222.

Page 92: Research from Dr. Ethan Kross: Ethan Kross, *Chatter* (New York: Crown, 2021), 19, 28, 39.

Page 93: When we procrastinate on a project, we do so in part because we are afraid to tackle it and afraid to fail: Procrastination isn't just reserved for fearsome experiences; we may also procrastinate on enjoyable ones. This is especially true when we feel we have an abundance of time. This explains why gift certificates often go unused (we assume we'll have time to redeem them in the future), and why so many of us do not visit our local museums and tourist sights, even though we might enjoy them (we live here, so we assume we can visit any time). For more information, see: Suzanne Shu and Ayelet Gneezy, "Procrastination of Enjoyable Experiences," *Journal of Marketing Research* 47, no. 5 (September 2009): http://dx .doi.org/10.2307/20751554.

Chapter 4

Page 99: Thinking can quickly turn into over-thinking: I first heard the term *overthinking* from Meredith Arthur, author of *Get Out of My Head* (New York: Running Press, 2020). According to Meredith, "overthinking is when preoccupied, cyclical thought patterns negatively impact your life emotionally and/or physically." When overthinking can't be tuned out and begins to interrupt our lives, we need to learn how to manage it.

Page 101: Psychological distancing is the process of zooming out from our worry to see the bigger picture: Kross, *Chatter*, 49.

Page 103: Think about which coping mechanisms pair best with the kinds of worries you encounter most often: These suggestions will be most helpful for those managing the day-to-day worries and anxieties of everyday life. If your anxiety is negatively interfering with your daily life, a licensed therapist can help you understand your anxiety and how to manage it. Depending on the severity and type of anxiety (generalized anxiety disorder, panic disorder, adjustment disorder, post-traumatic stress disorder, among others), your therapist may suggest a number of personalized steps to help.

Page 118: On the other hand, bright, colorful spaces leave us more alert and boost our energy: Ingrid Fetell, *Joyful* (New York: Little, Brown Spark, 2018), 23.

Page 118: Blues and greens are particularly restful; they help relieve stress and anxiety: Qing Li, *Forest Bathing* (New York, New York: Viking, 2018), 172.

Page 119: "Sound possesses a unique temporal nature": Lavender Suarez, *Transcendent Waves* (New York: Anthology Editions, 2020), 53.

Page 120: "Not every sound is a song, but any sound can be part of a song": Suarez, *Transcendent Waves*, 65.

Page 120: These sounds reduce our typically inward focus: Li, *Forest Bathing*, 164–165.

Page 120: Our strongest music memories are formed in our teens and early twenties: Suarez, *Transcendent Waves*, 17.

Page 121: Many of us crave silence but also find ourselves discomfited by it: In my first book, *Listen Like You Mean It* (New York: Portfolio, 2021), I note how this phenomenon occurs in conversation as well. In conversation, we refer to moments of silence as "awkward silence" and often take them as a sign that we've bored, offended, or made someone uncomfortable—when truthfully, it is often our own discomfort on display.

Page 127: The right kind of exercise can even quiet the part of the brain responsible for planning, analyzing, and critiquing: Annie Murphy Paul, *The Extended Mind* (Boston: Houghton Mifflin Harcourt, 2021), 53. "Intense" exercise is most helpful for quieting our planning brain. For example, running for forty minutes helps ideas and thoughts surface more freely; unrestrained by our rational, judging brain, we can let our creative thoughts run free.

Page 129: And walking benefits us physically too: Shane O'Mara, *In Praise of Walking* (New York: W. W. Norton & Company, 2020), 10–11.

Page 129: There is a reason that most of the great thinker-walkers we know of are men: For a look at non-male thinker-walkers, see Annabel Abbs, *Windswept* (Portland: Tin House, 2021), which chronicles the story of several women walkers throughout history, along with her own journey in walking. Cheryl Strayed's *Wild* (New York: Alfred A. Knopf, 2012) is another woman-walking narrative.

Page 131: Swimming is a proven mood booster, promotes relaxation, and is also helpful for anxiety: "Health Benefits of Swimming," *Centers for Disease Control and Prevention*, February 18, 2022, https://www.cdc.gov /healthywater/swimming/swimmers/health _benefits_water_exercise.html.

Page 131: "The body is engaged in full physical movement, but the mind itself floats, untethered": Bonnie Tsui, *Why We Swim* (Chapel Hill: Algonquin Books, 2020), 107–108; 233.

Page 132: In this space, "all that's being asked of you is to let go of 'doing'": Tracee Stanley, *Radiant Rest* (Boulder: Shambhala, 2021), 63.

Page 134: Physical touch has been shown to reduce blood pressure, heart rate, and the stress hormone cortisol: Tiffany Field, "Touch for Socioemotional and Physical Well-being: A Review," *Developmental Review* 30, no. 4 (December 2010): 367–383, https://doi.org /10.1016/j.dr.2011.01.001.

Page 134: It can also help with symptoms of anxiety: Mark Hyman Rapaport, Pamela J. Schettler, Erika R. Larson, Dedric Carroll, Margaret Sharenko, James Nettles, and Becky

Kinkead, "Massage Therapy for Psychiatric Disorders," *Focus* 16, no. 1 (Winter 2018): 24–31, https://doi.org/10.1176/appi.focus.20170043.

Page 134: Even petting a dog can be a positive bonding experience: Kerstin Uvnäs-Moberg, Linda Handlin, and Maria Petersson, "Self-soothing behaviors with particular reference to oxytocin release induced by non-noxious sensory stimulation." *Frontiers in Psychology* 5 (2014): 1529, https://doi.org/10.3389/fpsyg.2014.01529.

Page 135: We can self-soothe with a hand to our heart: Aljoscha Dreisoerner, Nina M. Junker, Wolff Schlotz, Julia Heimrich, Svenja Bloemeke, Beate Ditzen, and Rolf van Dick, "Self-soothing touch and being hugged reduce cortisol responses to stress: A randomized controlled trial on stress, physical touch, and social identity," *Comprehensive Psychoneuroendocrinology* 8 (November 2021): 100091, https://doi.org/10.1016/j.cpnec.2021.100091.

Page 138: This activates your parasympathetic response: Chloe Williams, "Cold Water Plunges Are Trendy. Can They Really Reduce Anxiety and Depression?," *New York Times*, February 20, 2022, https://www.nytimes.com/2022/02/20/well/mind/cold-water-plunge-mental-health.html This is also known as the mammalian dive reflex.

Page 139: According to the CDC, roughly seventy million American adults are chronically sleep-deprived: "About Our Program—Sleep and Sleep Disorders," *Centers For Disease Control and Prevention*, September 13, 2022, https://www.cdc.gov/sleep/about_us.html.

Page 143: As sleep researcher Dr. Matthew Walker puts it: Matthew Walker, *Why We Sleep* (New York: Scribner, 2017), 275.

Page 145: According to Daniel Pink: Daniel H. Pink, *When* (New York: Riverhead Books, 2018), 76.

Page 146: As journalist and coffee aficionado Michael Pollan puts it: Michael Pollan, *This Is Your Mind on Plants* (New York: Penguin Press, 2021), 95.

Page 149: "The basic idea is that a lot of times we learn who we are by observing what we do and say": Adam Grant, "Adam Grant Returns," interview by Dax Shepard and Monica Padman, *Armchair Expert*, February 4, 2021, 00:57:32 to 00:58:11, https://www.happyscribe.com/public/armchair-expert-with-dax-shepard/adam-grant-returns.

Page 152: Women experience hormonal changes every month: Jennifer Chen, "Women, Are Your Hormones Keeping You Up at Night?," *Yale Medicine*, July 10, 2017, https://www.yalemedicine.org/news/women-are-your-hormones-keeping-you-up-at-night.

Page 156: After exposure to nature, time feels expansive: Paul, *The Extended Mind*, 108.

Page 156: As psychologist Dr. Ethan Kross puts it: Kross, *Chatter*, 111.

Page 156: We feel more open, relaxed, and less time-pressured and impatient: Florence Williams, *The Nature Fix* (New York: W. W. Norton & Company, 2017), 200.

Page 157: It can aid in how quickly we make progress at school or recover from a hospital stay: Fetell, *Joyful*, 35.

Page 158: It helps to activate our parasympathetic (rest-and-digest) system: Qing Li, *Forest Bathing* (New York: Viking, 2018), 64.

Page 160: "Nature by the Dose" illustration: Based on research from Williams, *The Nature Fix*, 143–144.

Page 161: In fact, research shows that just *looking* at photos or videos of green spaces can be good for our well-being: Williams, *The Nature Fix*, 140.

Page 174: Music therapy, sand therapy, art therapy, dance and movement therapy, and even animal therapy can be helpful for processing trauma and treating stress and anxiety: For more on each of these, see:

Animal therapy: Arlin Cuncic, "What is Animal-Assisted Therapy (AAT)?," *Verywell Mind*, July 9, 2021, https://www.verywellmind.com/animal-assisted-therapy-for-social-anxiety-disorder-4049422.

Art therapy: "What is Art Therapy?,"
Kendra Cherry, *Verywell Mind*, August 31,
2021, https://www.verywellmind.com
/what-is-art-therapy-2795755.

Sand therapy: Amy Morin, "What is Sand
Tray Therapy?," *Verywell Mind*, August 29,
2021, https://www.verywellmind.com/what
-is-sand-tray-therapy-4589493.

Music therapy: Cathy Wong, "What is
Music Therapy?," *Verywell Mind*, July 14,
2021, https://www.verywellmind.com
/benefits-of-music-therapy-89829.

Dance therapy: Sara Lindberg, "What is
Dance Therapy?," *Verywell Mind*, July 9, 2021,
https://www.verywellmind.com/dance-therapy
-and-eating-disorder-treatment-5094952.

Page 175: Doodling, collaging, coloring books,
and playing with sand: "3 Reasons Adult
Coloring Can Actually Relax Your Brain,"
Cleveland Clinic, May 17, 2020, https://health
.clevelandclinic.org/3-reasons-adult-coloring
-can-actually-relax-brain/.

Eleanor Ainge Roy, "Colouring Books for
Adults Benefit Mental Health, Study Suggests,"
Guardian (UK edition), November 8, 2017,
https://www.theguardian.com/society/2017/nov
/09/colouring-books-for-adults-benefit-mental
-health-study-new-zealand-anxiety-depression.

Page 175: Having a social support network can
help: "Stress management and social support,"
Mayo Clinic, https://www.mayoclinic.org/healthy
-lifestyle/stress-management/in-depth/social
-support/art-20044445.

Chapter 5

Page 185: As author and therapist Nedra
Tawwab says: Tawwab, *Set Boundaries, Find
Peace: A Guide to Reclaiming Yourself*, 151.

Page 187: According to Nedra Tawwab:
Tawwab, *Set Boundaries, Find Peace: A Guide to
Reclaiming Yourself*, 114–115.

Page 190: These moments offer what
Milkman calls "psychological do-overs": Katy
Milkman, *How to Change* (New York: Portfolio,
2021), 22.

Page 191: One simple way of starting small:
James Clear, *Atomic Habits* (New York: Avery,
2018), 162.

Page 191: James Clear suggests: Clear calls
this an "implementation intention." Clear,
Atomic Habits, 71.

Page 192: Each action is a "vote" for the
person you want to become: Clear, *Atomic
Habits*, 39.

Page 193: "Close the gap between yourself and
your spirit": Maggie Smith, *Keep Moving* (New
York: Atria, 2020), 59.

Page 197: Yet research from social psychologist
Dr. Wendy Wood shows that strong intentions
and willpower can only take us so far: Wendy
Wood, *Good Habits, Bad Habits* (New York:
Farrar, Straus and Giroux, 2019), 17.

Page 199: This kind of thinking is not only
distracting but mentally taxing: Eldar and
Mullainathan, *Scarcity: The New Science of Having
Less and How It Defines Our Lives*, 217–218.

Page 199: We want to reduce what economist
Dr. Eldar Shafir and psychologist Dr. Sendhil
Mullainathan call vigilance choices: Eldar and
Mullainathan, *Scarcity: The New Science of Having
Less and How It Defines Our Lives*, 211.

Page 203: These techniques are particularly
useful for everyday evening recovery: Sabine
Sonnentag, Bonnie Hayden Cheng, and Stacey
L. Parker, "Recovery from Work: Advancing
the Field Toward the Future," *Annual Review
of Organizational Psychology and Organizational
Behavior* 9 (January 2022): 33–60, https://doi
.org/10.1146/annurev-orgpsych-012420-091355.

Page 203: Try "low-duty" activities:
Sonnentag, Cheng, and Parker, "Recovery
from Work," 33–60.

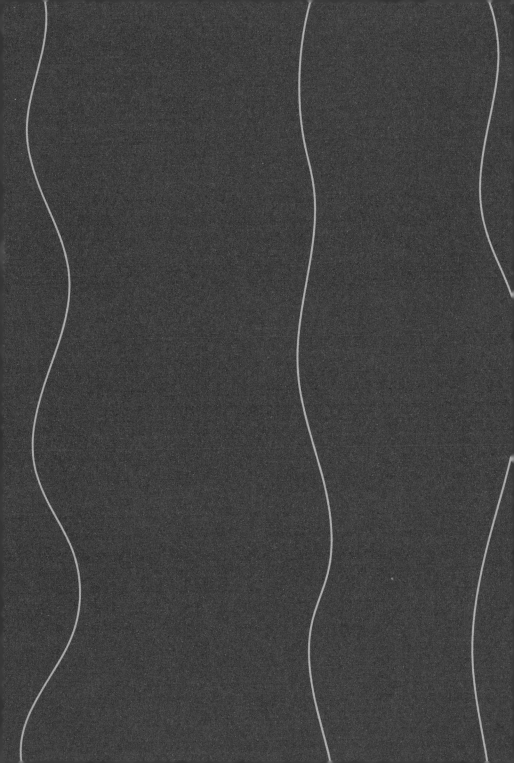